FREE

Free Study Tips DVD

In addition to the tips and content in this guide, we have created a FREE DVD with helpful study tips to further assist your exam preparation. **This FREE Study Tips DVD provides you with top-notch tips to conquer your exam and reach your goals.**

Our simple request in exchange for the strategy-packed DVD is that you email us your feedback about our study guide. We would love to hear what you thought about the guide, and we welcome any and all feedback—positive, negative, or neutral. It is our #1 goal to provide you with top-quality products and customer service.

To receive your **FREE Study Tips DVD**, email freedvd@apexprep.com. Please put "FREE DVD" in the subject line and put the following in the email:

a. The name of the study guide you purchased.

b. Your rating of the study guide on a scale of 1-5, with 5 being the highest score.

c. Any thoughts or feedback about your study guide.

d. Your first and last name and your mailing address, so we know where to send your free DVD!

Thank you!

The ATI TEAS Tutor

TEAS Study Guide 2020 & 2021 and Practice Test Questions for the Test of Essential Academic Skills [Updated for the 6th Edition]

APEX Test Prep

Table of Contents

Test Taking Strategies

1. Reading the Whole Question

A popular assumption in Western culture is the idea that we don't have enough time for anything. We speed while driving to work, we want to read an assignment for class as quickly as possible, or we want the line in the supermarket to dwindle faster. However, speeding through such events robs us from being able to thoroughly appreciate and understand what's happening around us. While taking a timed test, the feeling one might have while reading a question is to find the correct answer as quickly as possible. Although pace is important, don't let it deter you from reading the whole question. Test writers know how to subtly change a test question toward the end in various ways, such as adding a negative or changing focus. If the question has a passage, carefully read the whole passage as well before moving on to the questions. This will help you process the information in the passage rather than worrying about the questions you've just read and where to find them. A thorough understanding of the passage or question is an important way for test takers to be able to succeed on an exam.

2. Examining Every Answer Choice

Let's say we're at the market buying apples. The first apple we see on top of the heap may *look* like the best apple, but if we turn it over we can see bruising on the skin. We must examine several apples before deciding which apple is the best. Finding the correct answer choice is like finding the best apple. Although it's tempting to choose an answer that seems correct at first without reading the others, it's important to read each answer choice thoroughly before making a final decision on the answer. The aim of a test writer might be to get as close as possible to the correct answer, so watch out for subtle words that may indicate an answer is incorrect. Once the correct answer choice is selected, read the question again and the answer in response to make sure all your bases are covered.

3. Eliminating Wrong Answer Choices

Sometimes we become paralyzed when we are confronted with too many choices. Which frozen yogurt flavor is the tastiest? Which pair of shoes look the best with this outfit? What type of car will fill my needs as a consumer? If you are unsure of which answer would be the best to choose, it may help to use process of elimination. We use "filtering" all the time on sites such as eBay® or Craigslist® to eliminate the ads that are not right for us. We can do the same thing on an exam. Process of elimination is crossing out the answer choices we know for sure are wrong and leaving the ones that might be correct. It may help to cover up the incorrect answer choice. Covering incorrect choices is a psychological act that alleviates stress due to the brain being exposed to a smaller amount of information. Choosing between two answer choices is much easier than choosing between all of them, and you have a better chance of selecting the correct answer if you have less to focus on.

4. Sticking to the World of the Question

When we are attempting to answer questions, our minds will often wander away from the question and what it is asking. We begin to see answer choices that are true in the real world instead of true in the world of the question. It may be helpful to think of each test question as its own little world. This world may be different from ours. This world may know as a truth that the chicken came before the egg or may assert that two plus two equals five. Remember that, no matter what hypothetical nonsense may be in the question, assume it to be true. If the question states that the chicken came before the egg, then choose your answer based on that truth. Sticking to the world of the question means placing all of our biases and assumptions aside and relying on the question to guide us to the correct answer. If we are simply looking for answers that are correct based on our own judgment, then we may choose incorrectly. Remember an answer that is true does not necessarily answer the question.

5. Key Words

If you come across a complex test question that you have to read over and over again, try pulling out some key words from the question in order to understand what exactly it is asking. Key words may be words that surround the question, such as *main idea, analogous, parallel, resembles, structured,* or *defines.* The question may be asking for the main idea, or it may be asking you to define something. Deconstructing the sentence may also be helpful in making the question simpler before trying to answer it. This means taking the sentence apart and obtaining meaning in pieces, or separating the question from the foundation of the question. For example, let's look at this question:

> Given the author's description of the content of paleontology in the first paragraph, which of the following is most parallel to what it taught?

The question asks which one of the answers most *parallels* the following information: The *description* of paleontology in the first paragraph. The first step would be to see *how* paleontology is described in the first paragraph. Then, we would find an answer choice that parallels that description. The question seems complex at first, but after we deconstruct it, the answer becomes much more attainable.

6. Subtle Negatives

Negative words in question stems will be words such as *not, but, neither,* or *except.* Test writers often use these words in order to trick unsuspecting test takers into selecting the wrong answer—or, at least, to test their reading comprehension of the question. Many exams will feature the negative words in all caps (*which of the following is NOT an example*), but some questions will add the negative word seamlessly into the sentence. The following is an example of a subtle negative used in a question stem:

> According to the passage, which of the following is *not* considered to be an example of paleontology?

If we rush through the exam, we might skip that tiny word, *not,* inside the question, and choose an answer that is opposite of the correct choice. Again, it's important to read the question fully, and double check for any words that may negate the statement in any way.

7. Spotting the Hedges

The word "hedging" refers to language that remains vague or avoids absolute terminology. Absolute terminology consists of words like *always, never, all, every, just, only, none,* and *must.* Hedging refers to words like *seem, tend, might, most, some, sometimes, perhaps, possibly, probability,* and *often.* In some cases, we want to choose answer choices that use hedging and avoid answer choices that use absolute terminology. It's important to pay attention to what subject you are on and adjust your response accordingly.

8. Restating to Understand

Every now and then we come across questions that we don't understand. The language may be too complex, or the question is structured in a way that is meant to confuse the test taker. When you come across a question like this, it may be worth your time to rewrite or restate the question in your own words in order to understand it better. For example, let's look at the following complicated question:

> Which of the following words, if substituted for the word *parochial* in the first paragraph, would LEAST change the meaning of the sentence?

Let's restate the question in order to understand it better. We know that they want the word *parochial* replaced. We also know that this new word would "least" or "not" change the meaning of the sentence. Now let's try the sentence again:

> Which word could we replace with *parochial,* and it would not change the meaning?

Restating it this way, we see that the question is asking for a synonym. Now, let's restate the question so we can answer it better:

> Which word is a synonym for the word *parochial?*

Before we even look at the answer choices, we have a simpler, restated version of a complicated question.

9. Predicting the Answer

After you read the question, try predicting the answer *before* reading the answer choices. By formulating an answer in your mind, you will be less likely to be distracted by any wrong answer choices. Using predictions will also help you feel more confident in the answer choice you select. Once you've chosen your answer, go back and reread the question and answer choices to make sure you have the best fit. If you have no idea what the answer may be for a particular question, forego using this strategy.

10. Avoiding Patterns

One popular myth in grade school relating to standardized testing is that test writers will often put multiple-choice answers in patterns. A runoff example of this kind of thinking is that the most common answer choice is "C," with "B" following close behind. Or, some will advocate certain made-up word patterns that simply do not exist. Test writers do not arrange their correct answer choices in any kind of pattern; their choices are randomized. There may even be times where the correct answer choice will be the same letter for two or three questions in a row, but we have no way of knowing when or if this might happen. Instead of trying to figure out what choice the test writer probably set as being correct, focus on what the *best answer choice* would be out of the answers you are presented with. Use the tips above, general knowledge, and reading comprehension skills in order to best answer the question, rather than looking for patterns that do not exist.

FREE DVD OFFER

Achieving a high score on your exam depends not only on understanding the content, but also on understanding how to apply your knowledge and your command of test taking strategies. **Because your success is our primary goal, we offer a FREE Study Tips DVD. It provides top-notch test taking strategies to help you optimize your testing experience.**

Our simple request in exchange for the strategy-packed DVD is that you email us your feedback about our study guide.

To receive your **FREE Study Tips DVD**, email freedvd@apexprep.com. Please put "FREE DVD" in the subject line and put the following in the email:

    a. The name of the study guide you purchased.

    b. Your rating of the study guide on a scale of 1-5, with 5 being the highest score.

    c. Any thoughts or feedback about your study guide.

    d. Your first and last name and your mailing address, so we know where to send your free DVD!

ATI TEAS Overview

Function of the Test

The TEAS test is a standardized Test of Essential Academic Skills given by the Assessment Technologies Institute (ATI) Nursing Education. Those who want to be considered for admissions into nursing school or an allied health school must take the TEAS as part of an overall assessment of qualification for the program. The TEAS test is nationwide and offered in both the United States and Canada. The newest version of the TEAS is called the ATI TEAS.

The TEAS test is very important in determining admissions to nursing programs, although the preferred score by nursing schools varies. The TEAS can be taken by students wishing to be considered for a nursing or health program, or for professionals already in the industry who want to advance their certification.

Test Administration

The TEAS test is offered by ATI Testing in PSI testing centers or at nursing schools or allied health schools at least once a week all year round. You can determine where these centers are by visiting the PSI exam's website directly or through beginning registration through atitesting.com. Once you start your registration for the TEAS, you will be shown various testing locations to choose from by city and state, ranging from metropolitan cities to less-populated towns. Retaking the test is permitted, but the rules vary by school. Disability accommodations can be made available by contacting the testing administration site.

Test Format

Once you present your ID to the staff, you will have a seat in the testing area. The format of the exam can either be computerized or on paper. Keep in mind that proctors will be standing around the room to monitor for disruption. The proctor will provide you with a calculator and scratch paper.

Breaks will begin at the end of each section. Other than these breaks, the testing clock will not stop. The staff at the administration center ask that you raise your hand for any kind of issues with the test. The following table depicts the sections on the TEAS, the number of questions, and the time limit given for each section:

Subject	Questions	Time
Reading	53	64 minutes
Math	36	54 minutes
Science	53	63 minutes
English and Language Usage	28	28 minutes
Total	**170**	**209 minutes**

Scoring

Scores are available immediately after taking the online version of the test. For those who take the paper version of the test, ATI Nursing Education will process the scores within 48 hours of receiving the test. The scores will provide your total scores, the individual content scores, and which specific topic areas were missed. Nursing programs all have a different minimum of TEAS scores required for admission into the program, so you will have to check with the appropriate schools. Nursing programs typically look at the composite score listed at the top of the score report. The report will also show the national mean and the program mean—the national mean composite score is usually between a 65% and a 75%.

Recent/Future Developments

The ATI TEAS is the sixth version of the test and was released in August 2016. Calculators may now be used on the newest version of the test. The ATI TEAS is the same difficulty level but has slightly different topic areas than its predecessor. The English and Language Usage section has been reduced, with the elimination of the Earth Science subsection.

Reading

Key Ideas and Details

Summarizing a Complex Text

An important skill is the ability to read a complex text and then reduce its length and complexity by focusing on the key events and details. A **summary** is a shortened version of the original text, written by the reader in their own words. The summary should be shorter than the original text, and it must be thoughtfully formed to include critical points from the original text.

In order to effectively summarize a complex text, it's necessary to understand the original source and identify the major points covered. It may be helpful to outline the original text to get the big picture and avoid getting bogged down in the minor details. For example, a summary wouldn't include a statistic from the original source unless it was the major focus of the text. It's also important for readers to use their own words, yet retain the original meaning of the passage. The key to a good summary is emphasizing the main idea without changing the focus of the original information.

The more complex a text, the more difficult it can be to summarize. Readers must evaluate all points from the original source and then filter out what they feel are the less necessary details. Only the essential ideas should remain. The summary often mirrors the original text's organizational structure. For example, in a problem-solution text structure, the author typically presents readers with a problem and then develops solutions through the course of the text. An effective summary would likely retain this general structure, rephrasing the problem and then reporting the most useful or plausible solutions.

Paraphrasing is somewhat similar to summarizing. It calls for the reader to take a small part of the passage and list or describe its main points. Paraphrasing is more than rewording the original passage, though. Like summary, it should be written in the reader's own words, while still retaining the meaning of the original source. The main difference between summarizing and paraphrasing is that a summary would be appropriate for a much larger text, while paraphrase might focus on just a few lines of text. Effective paraphrasing will indicate an understanding of the original source, yet still help the reader expand on their interpretation. A paraphrase should neither add new information nor remove essential facts that change the meaning of the source.

Inferring the Logical Conclusion from a Reading Selection

Making an inference from a selection means to make an educated guess from the passage read. **Inferences** should be conclusions based off of sound evidence and reasoning. When multiple-choice test questions ask about the logical conclusion that can be drawn from reading text, the test-taker must identify which choice will unavoidably lead to that conclusion. In order to eliminate the incorrect choices, the test-taker should come up with a hypothetical situation wherein an answer choice is true, but the conclusion is not true.

For example, here is an example with three answer choices:

Fred purchased the newest PC available on the market. Therefore, he purchased the most expensive PC in the computer store.

What can one assume for this conclusion to follow logically?

a. Fred enjoys purchasing expensive items.
b. PCs are some of the most expensive personal technology products available.
c. The newest PC is the most expensive one.

The premise of the text is the first sentence: Fred purchased the newest PC. The conclusion is the second sentence: Fred purchased the most expensive PC. Recent release and price are two different factors; the difference between them is the logical gap. To eliminate the gap, one must equate whatever new information the conclusion introduces with the pertinent information the premise has stated. This example simplifies the process by having only one of each: one must equate product recency with product price. Therefore, a possible bridge to the logical gap could be a sentence stating that the newest PCs always cost the most.

Identifying the Topic, Main Idea, and Supporting Details

The **topic** of a text is the general subject matter. Text topics can usually be expressed in one word, or a few words at most. Additionally, readers should ask themselves what point the author is trying to make. This point is the **main idea** of the text, the one thing the author wants readers to know concerning the topic. Once the author has established the main idea, they will support the main idea by supporting details. **Supporting details** are evidence that support the main idea and include personal testimonies, examples, or statistics.

One analogy for these components and their relationships is that a text is like a well-designed house. The topic is the roof, covering all rooms. The main idea is the frame. The supporting details are the various rooms. To identify the topic of a text, readers can ask themselves what or who the author is writing about in the paragraph. To locate the main idea, readers can ask themselves what one idea the author wants readers to know about the topic. To identify supporting details, readers can put the main idea into question form and ask "what does the author use to prove or explain their main idea?"

Let's look at an example. An author is writing an essay about the Amazon rainforest and trying to convince the audience that more funding should go into protecting the area from deforestation. The author makes the argument stronger by including evidence of the benefits of the rainforest: it provides habitats to a variety of species, it provides much of the earth's oxygen which in turn cleans the atmosphere, and it is the home to medicinal plants that may be the answer to some of the world's deadliest diseases.

Here is an outline of the essay looking at topic, main idea, and supporting details:

Topic: Amazon rainforest
Main Idea: The Amazon rainforest should receive more funding in order to protect it from deforestation.
Supporting Details:
    1. It provides habitats to a variety of species
    2. It provides much of the earth's oxygen which in turn cleans the atmosphere
    3. It is home to medicinal plants that may be the answer to some of the world's deadliest diseases.

Notice that the topic of the essay is listed in a few key words: "Amazon rainforest". The main idea tells us what about the topic is important: that the topic should be funded in order to prevent deforestation. Finally, the supporting details are what author relies on to convince the audience to act or to believe in the truth of the main idea.

Following a Given Set of Directions

To follow directions, an individual must hold them in short-term memory while using working memory and language to comprehend the information. Certain word types are found more often than others in directions; these include adjectives, negatives, conjunctions, and prepositions. Understanding the concepts that these word types represent is important, especially in academics. For example, the CELF (Clinical Evaluation of Language Fundamentals) subtest on Concepts and Following Directions is one of most frequently administered assessment instruments for evaluating how well people follow directions, and almost every item on this subtest combines negatives, conjunctions, and prepositions. Being able to follow a direction requires understanding of the direction's specific words. Even single-step directions can be challenging, especially when they contain negatives ("Do *not* circle the even-numbered items"). In addition to language comprehension, the ability to follow directions requires interest in the activity, motivation to follow the directions, and paying attention to the directions.

Basic one-step directions use simple syntax and kid's earliest learned words, like the following:

- Give me the cup
- Tie your shoe
- Say your name
- Close the door
- Throw that away

Expanded one-step directions add a few negatives, contractions, and slightly more advanced vocabulary, like the following:

- Don't touch the blue one
- Show me which one is not yellow
- Use the bigger pen
- Throw all of your trash away
- Take out your small, green notebook

Basic two-step directions include one basic conjunction, or one added phrase, like the following:

- Take off your socks and put them in the hamper
- Close the door and then sit down

- Write your name on the test before beginning
- Give me the glass that is empty

Expanded two-step directions have a structure added to two steps, like the following:

Throw your partner's trash away before you start the assignment

Complex directions include vocabulary and syntax that develop later, plus multiple clauses, like the following:

Please turn off all cell phones after you have taken your seats

The following example shows why it's extremely important to read all the directions in a test setting first before acting on any of them. Follow the directions below:

1. Carefully read everything in the directions before you do anything.
2. Write your name on the top of this page.
3. Put your birthday and date underneath your name.
4. Write an "Z" on an empty space anywhere on the page.
5. Circle the "Z" and draw a line below it referring to "Y."
6. Draw a line from "Y" referring to "X."
7. Draw a box at the bottom of this page.
8. Describe the shape you drew around the letters inside the box.
9. Write your name inside the box.
10. Now that you've carefully read everything, follow only directions (1) and (2).

Those who get to direction 10 without having acted on any instructions yet will save a lot of wasted time opposed to those who immediately begin to act on the instructions. Remember, read all the directions before you begin, and you will have a better idea of what the bigger picture entails!

Identifying Specific Information from a Printed Communication

Business Memos
Whereas everyday office memos were traditionally typed on paper, photocopied, and distributed, today they are more often typed on computers and distributed via e-mail, both interoffice and externally. Technology has thus made these communications more immediate. It is also helpful for people to read carefully and be familiar with memo components. For example, e-mails automatically provide the same "To:, From:, and Re:" lines traditionally required in paper memos, and in corresponding places—the top of the page/screen. Readers should observe whether "To: names/positions" include all intended recipients in case of misdirection errors or omitted recipients. "From:" informs sender level, role, and who will receive responses when people click "Reply." Users must be careful not to click "Reply All" unintentionally. They should also observe the "CC:" line, typically below "Re:," showing additional recipients.

Classified Ads
Classified advertisements include "Help Wanted" ads informing readers of positions open for hiring, real estate listings, cars for sale, and home and business services available. Traditional ads in newspapers had to save space, and this necessity has largely transferred to online ads. Because of needing to save space, advertisers employ many abbreviations. For example, here are some examples of abbreviations:

- FT=full-time
- PT=part-time

- A/P=accounts payable
- A/R=accounts receivable
- Asst.=assistant
- Bkkg.=bookkeeping
- Comm.=commission
- Bet.=between
- EOE=equal opportunity employer
- G/L=general ledger
- Immed.=immediately
- Exc.=excellent
- Exp.=experience
- Eves.=evenings
- Secy.=secretary
- Temp=temporary
- Sal=salary
- Req=required
- Refs=references
- Wk=week or work
- WPM=words per minute

Classified ads frequently use abbreviations to take up less space, both on paper and digitally on websites. Those who read these ads will find it less confusing if they learn some common abbreviations used by businesses when advertising job positions. Here are some examples:

- Mgt.=management
- Mgr.=manager
- Mfg.=manufacturing
- Nat'l=national
- Dept.=department
- Min.=minimum
- Yrs.=years
- Nec=necessary
- Neg=negotiable
- Oppty=opportunity
- O/T=overtime
- K=1,000

Readers of classified ads may focus on certain features to the exclusion of others. For example, if a reader sees the job title or salary they are seeking, or notices the experience, education, degree, or other credentials required match their own qualifications perfectly, they may fail to notice other important information, like "No benefits." This is important because the employers are disclosing that they will not provide health insurance, retirement accounts, paid sick leave, paid maternity/paternity leave, paid vacation, etc. to any employee whom they hire. Someone expecting a traditional 9 to 5 job who fails to observe that an ad states "Evenings" or just the abbreviation "Eves" will be disappointed, as will the applicant who overlooks a line saying "Some evenings and weekends reqd." Applicants overlooking information like "Apply in person" may e-mail or mail their resumes and receive no response. The job hopeful with no previous experience and one reference must attend to information like "Minimum 5 yrs. exp, 3 refs," meaning they likely will not qualify.

Employment Ads

Job applicants should pay attention to the information included in classified employment ads. On one hand, they do need to believe and accept certain statements, such as "Please, no phone calls," which is frequently used by employers posting ads on Craigslist and similar websites. New applicants just graduated from or still in college will be glad to see "No exp necessary" in some ads, indicating they need no previous work experience in that job category. "FT/PT" means the employer offers the options of working full-time or part-time, another plus for students. On the other hand, ad readers should also take into consideration the fact that many employers list all the attributes of their *ideal* employee, but they do not necessarily expect to find such a candidate. If a potential applicant's education, training, credentials, and experience are not exactly the same as what the employer lists as desired but are not radically different either, it can be productive to apply anyway, while honestly representing one's actual qualifications.

Atlases

A road atlas is a publication designed to assist travelers who are driving on road trips rather than taking airplanes, trains, ships, etc. Travelers use road atlases to determine which routes to take and places to stop; how to navigate specific cities, locate landmarks, estimate mileages and travel times; see photographs of places they plan to visit; and find other travel-related information. One familiar, reputable road atlas is published by the National Geographic Society. It includes detailed, accurate maps of the United States, Canada, and Mexico; historic sites, scenic routes, recreation information, and points of interest; and its Adventure Edition spotlights 100 top U.S. adventure destinations and most popular national parks. The best-selling road atlas in the United States, also probably the best-known and most trusted, is published annually by Rand McNally, which has published road atlases for many years. It includes maps, mileage charts, information on tourism and road construction, maps of individual city details, and the editor's favorite road trips (in the 2016 edition) including recommended points of interest en route.

Owners' Manuals

An owner's manual is typically a booklet, but may also be as short as a page or as long as a book, depending on the individual instance. The purpose of an owner's manual is to give the owner instructions, usually step-by-step, for how to use a specific product or a group or range of products. Manuals accompany consumer products as diverse as cars, computers, tablets, smartphones, printers, home appliances, shop machines, and many others. In addition to directions for operating products, they include important warnings of things *not* to do that pose safety or health hazards or can damage the product and void the manufacturer's product warranty, like immersion in water, exposure to high temperatures, operating something for too long, dropping fragile items, or rough handling. Manuals teach correct operating practices, sequences, precautions, and cautions, averting many costly and/or dangerous mishaps.

Food Labels

When reading the labels on food products, it is often necessary to interpret the nutrition facts and other product information. Without the consumer's being aware and informed of this, much of this information can be very misleading. For example, a popular brand name of corn chips lists the calories, fat, etc. per serving in the nutrition facts printed on the bag, but on closer inspection, it defines a serving size as six chips—far fewer than most people would consume at a time. Serving sizes and the number of servings per container can be unrealistic. For example, a jumbo muffin's wrapper indicates it contains three servings. Not only do most consumers not divide a muffin and eat only part; but it is moreover rather difficult to cut a muffin into equal thirds. A king-sized package of chili cheese-flavored corn chips says it contains 4.5 servings per container. This is not very useful information, since people cannot divide the package into equal servings and are unlikely to eat four servings and then ½ a serving.

Product Packaging
Consumers today cannot take product labels at face value. While many people do not read or even look at the information on packages before eating their contents, those who do must use more consideration and analysis than they might expect to understand it. For example, a well-known brand of strawberry-flavored breakfast toaster pastry displays a picture of four whole strawberries on the wrapper. While this looks appealing, encouraging consumers to infer the product contains wholesome fruit—and perhaps even believe it contains four whole strawberries—reading the ingredients list reveals it contains only 2 percent or less of dried strawberries. A consumer must be detail-oriented (and curious or motivated enough) to read the full ingredients list, which also reveals unhealthy corn syrup and high fructose corn syrup high on the list after enriched flour. Consumers must also educate themselves about euphemistically misleading terms: "enriched" flour has vitamins and minerals added, but it is refined flour without whole grain, bran, or fiber.

While manufacturers generally provide extensive information printed on their package labels, it is typically in very small print—many consumers do not read it—and even consumers who do read all the information must look for small details to discover that the information is often not realistic. For example, a box of brownie mix lists grams of fat, total calories, and calories from fat. However, by paying attention to small details like asterisks next to this information, and finding the additional information referenced by the asterisks, the consumer discovers that these amounts are for only the dry mix—not the added eggs, oil, or milk. Consumers typically do not eat dry cake mixes, and having to determine and add the fat and calories from the additional ingredients is inconvenient. In another example, a box of macaroni and cheese mix has an asterisk by the fat grams indicating these are for the macaroni only without the cheese, butter, or milk required, which contributes 6.4 times more fat.

Ingredients' Lists
Consumers can realize the importance of reading drug labeling through an analogy: What might occur if they were to read only part of the directions on a standardized test? Reading only part of the directions on medications can have similar, even more serious consequences. Prescription drug packages typically contain inserts, which provide extremely extensive, thorough, detailed information, including results of clinical trials and statistics showing patient responses and adverse effects. Some over-the-counter medications include inserts, and some do not. "Active ingredients" are those ingredients making medication effective. "Inactive ingredients" including flavorings, preservatives, stabilizers, and emulsifiers have purposes, but not to treat symptoms. "Uses" indicates which symptoms a medication is meant to treat. "Directions" tell the dosage, frequency, maximum daily amount, and other requirements, like "Take with food," "Do not operate heavy machinery while using," etc. Drug labels also state how to store the product, like at what temperature or away from direct sunlight or humidity.

Many drugs which were previously available only by doctor prescription have recently become available over the counter without a prescription. While enough years of testing may have determined that these substances typically do not cause serious problems, consumers must nevertheless thoroughly read and understand all the information on the labels before taking them. If they do not, they could still suffer serious harm. For example, some individuals have allergies to specific substances. Both prescription and over-the-counter medication products list their ingredients, including warnings about allergies. Allergic reactions can include anaphylactic shock, which can be fatal if not treated immediately. Also, consumers must read and follow dosing directions: taking more than directed can cause harm, and taking less can be ineffective to treat symptoms. Some medication labels warn not to mix them with certain other drugs to avoid harmful drug interactions. Additionally, without reading ingredients, some consumers take multiple products including the same active ingredients, resulting in overdoses.

Identifying Information from a Graphic Representation of Information

Line Graphs

Line graphs are useful for visually representing data that vary continuously over time, like an individual student's test scores. The horizontal or *x*-axis shows dates/times; the vertical or *y*-axis shows point values. A dot is plotted on the point where each horizontal date line intersects each vertical number line, and then these dots are connected, forming a line. Line graphs show whether changes in values over time exhibit trends like ascending, descending, flat, or more variable, like going up and down at different times. For example, suppose a student's scores on the same type of reading test were 75% in October, 80% in November, 78% in December, 82% in January, 85% in February, 88% in March, and 90% in April. A line graph of these scores would look like this.

Bar Graphs

Bar graphs feature equally spaced, horizontal or vertical rectangular bars representing numerical values. They can show change over time as line graphs do, but unlike line graphs, bar graphs can also show differences and similarities among values at a single point in time. Bar graphs are also helpful for visually representing data from different categories, especially when the horizontal axis displays some value that is not numerical, like basketball players with their heights:

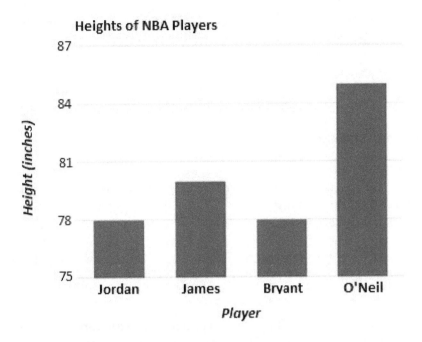

Heights of NBA Players

Pie Charts
Pie charts, also called **circle graphs**, are good for representing percentages or proportions of a whole quantity because they represent the whole as a circle or "pie", with the various proportion values shown as "slices" or wedges of the pie. This gives viewers a clear idea of how much of a total each item occupies. For example, biologists may have information that 62% of dogs have brown eyes, 20% have green eyes, and 18% have blue eyes. A pie chart of these distributions would look like this:

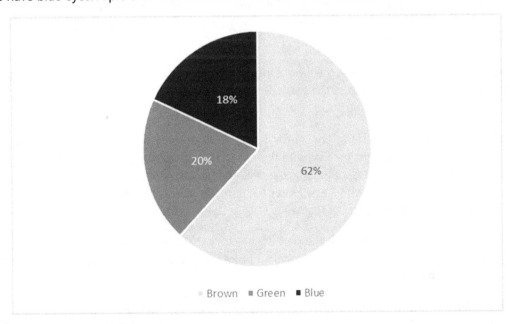

Pictograms
Magazines, newspapers, and other similar publications designed for consumption by the general public often use pictograms to represent data. **Pictograms** feature icons or symbols that look like whatever

category of data is being counted, like little silhouettes shaped like human beings commonly used to represent people. If the data involve large numbers, like populations, one person symbol might represent one million people, or one thousand, etc. For smaller values, such as how many individuals out of ten fit a given description, one symbol might equal one person. Male and female silhouettes are used to differentiate gender, and child shapes for children. Little clock symbols are used to represent amounts of time, such as a given number of hours; calendar pages might depict months; suns and moons could show days and nights; hourglasses might represent minutes. While pictogram symbols are easily recognizable and appealing to general viewers, one disadvantage is that it is difficult to display partial symbols for in-between quantities.

Recognizing Events in a Sequence

Sequence structure is the order of events in which a story or information is presented to the audience. Sometimes the text will be presented in chronological order, or sometimes it will be presented by displaying the most recent information first, then moving backwards in time. The sequence structure depends on the author, the context, and the audience. The structure of a text also depends on the genre in which the text is written. Is it literary fiction? Is it a magazine article? Is it instructions for how to complete a certain task? Different genres will have different purposes for switching up the sequence of their writing.

Narrative Structure

The structure presented in literary fiction is also known as **narrative structure**. Narrative structure is the foundation on which the text moves. The basic ways for moving the text along are in the plot and the setting. The plot is the sequence of events in the narrative that move the text forward through cause and effect. The setting of a story is the place or time period in which the story takes place. Narrative structure has two main categories: linear and nonlinear.

Linear Narrative

Linear narrative is a narrative told in chronological order. Traditional linear narratives will follow the plot diagram below depicting the narrative arc. The narrative arc consists of the exposition, conflict, rising action, climax, falling action, and resolution.

- Exposition: The exposition is in the beginning of a narrative and introduces the characters, setting, and background information of the story. The importance of the exposition lies in its framing of the upcoming narrative. Exposition literally means "a showing forth" in Latin.

- Conflict: The conflict, in a traditional narrative, is presented toward the beginning of the story after the audience becomes familiar with the characters and setting. The conflict is a single instance between characters, nature, or the self, in which the central character is forced to make a decision or move forward with some kind of action. The conflict presents something for the main character, or **protagonist**, to overcome.

- Rising Action: The rising action is the part of the story that leads into the climax. The rising action will feature the development of characters and plot, and creates the tension and suspense that eventually lead to the climax.

- Climax: The climax is the part of the story where the tension produced in the rising action comes to a culmination. The climax is the peak of the story. In a traditional structure, everything before the climax builds up to it, and everything after the climax falls from it. It is the height of the narrative, and is usually either the most exciting part of the story or is marked by some turning point in the character's journey.

- Falling Action: The falling action happens as a result of the climax. Characters continue to develop, although there is a wrapping up of loose ends here. The falling action leads to the resolution.

- Resolution: The resolution is where the story comes to an end and usually leaves the reader with the satisfaction of knowing what happened within the story and why. However, stories do not always end in this fashion. Sometimes readers can be confused or frustrated at the end from lack of information or the absence of a happy ending.

Nonlinear Narrative

A **nonlinear narrative** deviates from the traditional narrative in that it does not always follow the traditional plot structure of the narrative arc. Nonlinear narratives may include structures that are disjointed, circular, or disruptive, in the sense that they do not follow chronological order, but rather a nontraditional order of structure. *In medias res* is an example of a structure that predates the linear narrative. ***In medias res*** is Latin for "in the middle of things," which is how many ancient texts, especially epic poems, began their story, such as Homer's *Iliad*. Instead of having a clear exposition with a full development of characters, they would begin right in the middle of the action.

Modernist texts in the late nineteenth and early twentieth century are known for their experimentation with disjointed narratives, moving away from traditional linear narrative. Disjointed narratives are depicted in novels like *Catch 22*, where the author, Joseph Heller, structures the narrative based on free association of ideas rather than chronology. Another nonlinear narrative can be seen in the novel *Wuthering Heights*, written by Emily Bronte, which disrupts the chronological order by being told retrospectively after the first chapter. There seem to be two narratives in *Wuthering Heights* working at the same time: a present narrative as well as a past narrative. Authors employ disrupting narratives for various reasons; some use it for the purpose of creating situational irony for the readers, while some use it to create a certain effect in the reader, such as excitement, or even a feeling of discomfort or fear.

Sequence Structure in Technical Documents

The purpose of technical documents, such as instructions manuals, cookbooks, or "user-friendly" documents, is to provide information to users as clearly and efficiently as possible. In order to do this, the sequence structure in technical documents that should be used is one that is as straightforward as possible. This usually involves some kind of chronological order or a direct sequence of events. For example, someone who is reading an instruction manual on how to set up their Smart TV wants directions in a clear, simple, straightforward manner that does not leave the reader to guess at the proper sequence or lead to confusion.

Sequence Structure in Informational Texts

The structure in informational texts depends again on the genre. For example, a newspaper article may start by stating an exciting event that happened, and then move on to talk about that event in chronological order, known as **sequence** or **order structure**. Many informational texts also use **cause and effect structure**, which describes an event and then identifies reasons for why that event occurred. Some essays may write about their subjects by way of **comparison and contrast**, which is a structure that compares two things or contrasts them to highlight their differences. Other documents, such as proposals, will have a **problem to solution structure**, where the document highlights some kind of problem and then offers a solution toward the end. Finally, some informational texts are written with lush details and description in order to captivate the audience, allowing them to visualize the information presented to them. This type of structure is known as **descriptive.**

Craft and Structure

Distinguishing Between Fact and Opinion, Biases, and Stereotypes

Facts and Opinions

A **fact** is a statement that is true empirically or an event that has actually occurred in reality, and can be proven or supported by evidence; it is generally objective. In contrast, an **opinion** is subjective, representing something that someone believes rather than something that exists in the absolute. People's individual understandings, feelings, and perspectives contribute to variations in opinion. Though facts are typically objective in nature, in some instances, a statement of fact may be both factual and yet also subjective. For example, emotions are individual subjective experiences. If an individual says that they feel happy or sad, the feeling is subjective, but the statement is factual; hence, it is a subjective fact. In contrast, if one person tells another that the other is feeling happy or sad—whether this is true or not—that is an assumption or an opinion.

Biases

Biases usually occur when someone allows their personal preferences or ideologies to interfere with what should be an objective decision. In personal situations, someone is biased towards someone if they favor them in an unfair way. In academic writing, being biased in your sources means leaving out objective information that would turn the argument one way or the other. The evidence of bias in academic writing makes the text less credible, so be sure to present all viewpoints when writing, not just your own, so to avoid coming off as biased. Being objective when presenting information or dealing with people usually allows the person to gain more credibility.

Stereotypes

Stereotypes are preconceived notions that place a particular rule or characteristics on an entire group of people. Stereotypes are usually offensive to the group they refer to or allies of that group, and often have negative connotations. The reinforcement of stereotypes isn't always obvious. Sometimes stereotypes can be very subtle and are still widely used in order for people to understand categories within the world. For example, saying that women are more emotional and intuitive than men is a stereotype, although this is still an assumption used by many in order to understand the differences between one another.

Recognizing the Structure of Texts in Various Formats

Text structure is the way in which the author organizes and presents textual information so readers can follow and comprehend it. One kind of text structure is sequence. This means the author arranges the text in a logical order from beginning to middle to end. There are three types of sequences:

- Chronological: ordering events in time from earliest to latest

- Spatial: describing objects, people, or spaces according to their relationships to one another in space

- Order of Importance: addressing topics, characters, or ideas according to how important they are, from either least important to most important

Chronological sequence is the most common sequential text structure. Readers can identify sequential structure by looking for words that signal it, like *first, earlier, meanwhile, next, then, later, finally;* and specific times and dates the author includes as chronological references.

Problem-Solution Text Structure

The problem-solution text structure organizes textual information by presenting readers with a problem and then developing its solution throughout the course of the text. The author may present a variety of alternatives as possible solutions, eliminating each as they are found unsuccessful, or gradually leading up to the ultimate solution. For example, in fiction, an author might write a murder mystery novel and have the character(s) solve it through investigating various clues or character alibis until the killer is identified. In nonfiction, an author writing an essay or book on a real-world problem might discuss various alternatives and explain their disadvantages or why they would not work before identifying the best solution. For scientific research, an author reporting and discussing scientific experiment results would explain why various alternatives failed or succeeded.

Comparison-Contrast Text Structure

Comparison identifies similarities between two or more things. **Contrast** identifies differences between two or more things. Authors typically employ both to illustrate relationships between things by highlighting their commonalities and deviations. For example, a writer might compare Windows and Linux as operating systems, and contrast Linux as free and open-source vs. Windows as proprietary. When writing an essay, sometimes it is useful to create an image of the two objects or events you are comparing or contrasting. Venn diagrams are useful because they show the differences as well as the similarities between two things. Once you've seen the similarities and differences on paper, it might be helpful to create an outline of the essay with both comparison and contrast. Every outline will look different, because every two or more things will have a different number of comparisons and contrasts. Say you are trying to compare and contrast carrots with sweet potatoes.

Here is an example of a compare/contrast outline using those topics:

- Introduction: Talk about why you are comparing and contrasting carrots and sweet potatoes. Give the thesis statement.
- Body paragraph 1: Sweet potatoes and carrots are both root vegetables (similarity)
- Body paragraph 2: Sweet potatoes and carrots are both orange (similarity)

- Body paragraph 3: Sweet potatoes and carrots have different nutritional components (difference)
- Conclusion: Restate the purpose of your comparison/contrast essay.

Of course, if there is only one similarity between your topics and two differences, you will want to rearrange your outline. Always tailor your essay to what works best with your topic.

Descriptive Text Structure

Description can be both a type of text structure and a type of text. Some texts are descriptive throughout entire books. For example, a book may describe the geography of a certain country, state, or region, or tell readers all about dolphins by describing many of their characteristics. Many other texts are not descriptive throughout, but use descriptive passages within the overall text. The following are a few examples of descriptive text:

- When the author describes a character in a novel
- When the author sets the scene for an event by describing the setting
- When a biographer describes the personality and behaviors of a real-life individual
- When a historian describes the details of a particular battle within a book about a specific war
- When a travel writer describes the climate, people, foods, and/or customs of a certain place

A hallmark of description is using sensory details, painting a vivid picture so readers can imagine it almost as if they were experiencing it personally.

Cause and Effect Text Structure

When using cause and effect to extrapolate meaning from text, readers must determine the cause when the author only communicates effects. For example, if a description of a child eating an ice cream cone includes details like beads of sweat forming on the child's face and the ice cream dripping down her hand faster than she can lick it off, the reader can infer or conclude it must be hot outside. A useful technique for making such decisions is wording them in "*If...then*" form, e.g. "*If* the child is perspiring and the ice cream melting, *then* it may be a hot day." Cause and effect text structures explain why certain events or actions resulted in particular outcomes. For example, an author might describe America's historical large flocks of dodo birds, the fact that gunshots did not startle/frighten dodos, and that because dodos did not flee, settlers killed whole flocks in one hunting session, explaining how the dodo was hunted into extinction.

Interpreting the Meaning of Words and Phrases Using Context

When readers encounter an unfamiliar word in text, they can use the surrounding **context**—the overall subject matter, specific chapter/section topic, and especially the immediate sentence context. Among others, one category of context clues is grammar. For example, the position of a word in a sentence and its relationship to the other words can help the reader establish whether the unfamiliar word is a verb, a noun, an adjective, an adverb, etc. This narrows down the possible meanings of the word to one part of speech. However, this may be insufficient. In a sentence that many birds *migrate* twice yearly, the reader can determine the word is a verb, and probably does not mean eat or drink; but it could mean travel, mate, lay eggs, hatch, molt, etc.

Some words can have a number of different meanings depending on how they are used. For example, the word *fly* has a different meaning in each of the following sentences:

- "His trousers have a fly on them."
- "He swatted the fly on his trousers."

- "Those are some fly trousers."
- "They went fly fishing."
- "She hates to fly."
- "If humans were meant to fly, they would have wings."

As strategies, readers can try substituting a familiar word for an unfamiliar one and see whether it makes sense in the sentence. They can also identify other words in a sentence, offering clues to an unfamiliar word's meaning.

Denotation and Connotation

Denotation refers to a word's explicit definition, like that found in the dictionary. Denotation is often set in comparison to connotation. **Connotation** is the emotional, cultural, social, or personal implication associated with a word. Denotation is more of an objective definition, whereas connotation can be more subjective, although many connotative meanings of words are similar for certain cultures. The denotative meanings of words are usually based on facts, and the connotative meanings of words are usually based on emotion. Here are some examples of words and their denotative and connotative meanings in Western culture:

Word	Denotative Meaning	Connotative Meaning
Home	A permanent place where one lives, usually as a member of a family.	A place of warmth; a place of familiarity; comforting; a place of safety and security. "Home" usually has a positive connotation.
Snake	A long reptile with no limbs and strong jaws that moves along the ground; some snakes have a poisonous bite.	An evil omen; a slithery creature (human or nonhuman) that is deceitful or unwelcome. "Snake" usually has a negative connotation.
Winter	A season of the year that is the coldest, usually from December to February in the northern hemisphere and from June to August in the southern hemisphere.	Circle of life, especially that of death and dying; cold or icy; dark and gloomy; hibernation, sleep, or rest. Winter can have a negative connotation, although many who have access to heat may enjoy the snowy season from their homes.

Evaluating the Author's Purpose in a Given Text

Authors may have many purposes for writing a specific text. Their purposes may be to try and convince readers to agree with their position on a subject, to impart information, or to entertain. Other writers are motivated to write from a desire to express their own feelings. Authors' purposes are their reasons for writing something. A single author may have one overriding purpose for writing or multiple reasons. An author may explicitly state their intention in the text, or the reader may need to infer that intention. Those who read reflectively benefit from identifying the purpose because it enables them to analyze information in the text. By knowing why the author wrote the text, readers can glean ideas for how to approach it.

The following is a list of questions readers can ask in order to discern an author's purpose for writing a text:

- From the title of the text, why do you think the author wrote it?
- Was the purpose of the text to give information to readers?
- Did the author want to describe an event, issue, or individual?
- Was it written to express emotions and thoughts?
- Did the author want to convince readers to consider a particular issue?
- Was the author primarily motivated to write the text to entertain?
- Why do you think the author wrote this text from a certain point of view?
- What is your response to the text as a reader?
- Did the author state their purpose for writing it?

Students should read to interpret information rather than simply content themselves with roles as text consumers. Being able to identify an author's purpose efficiently improves reading comprehension, develops critical thinking, and makes students more likely to consider issues in depth before accepting writer viewpoints. Authors of fiction frequently write to entertain readers. Another purpose for writing fiction is making a political statement; for example, Jonathan Swift wrote "A Modest Proposal" (1729) as a political satire. Another purpose for writing fiction as well as nonfiction is to persuade readers to take some action or further a particular cause. Fiction authors and poets both frequently write to evoke certain moods; for example, Edgar Allan Poe wrote novels, short stories, and poems that evoke moods of gloom, guilt, terror, and dread. Another purpose of poets is evoking certain emotions: love is popular, as in Shakespeare's sonnets and numerous others. In "The Waste Land" (1922), T.S. Eliot evokes society's alienation, disaffection, sterility, and fragmentation.

Authors seldom directly state their purposes in texts. Some students may be confronted with nonfiction texts such as biographies, histories, magazine and newspaper articles, and instruction manuals, among others. To identify the purpose in nonfiction texts, students can ask the following questions:

- Is the author trying to teach something?
- Is the author trying to persuade the reader?
- Is the author imparting factual information only?
- Is this a reliable source?
- Does the author have some kind of hidden agenda?

To apply author purpose in nonfictional passages, students can also analyze sentence structure, word choice, and transitions to answer the aforementioned questions and to make inferences. For example, authors wanting to convince readers to view a topic negatively often choose words with negative connotations.

Narrative Writing
Narrative writing tells a story. The most prominent examples of narrative writing are fictional novels. Here are some examples:

- Mark Twain's The Adventures of Tom Sawyer and The Adventures of Huckleberry Finn
- Victor Hugo's *Les Misérables*
- Charles Dickens' Great Expectations, David Copperfield, and A Tale of Two Cities
- Jane Austen's Northanger Abbey, Mansfield Park, Pride and Prejudice, Sense and Sensibility, and Emma

- Toni Morrison's Beloved, The Bluest Eye, and Song of Solomon
- Gabriel García Márquez's One Hundred Years of Solitude and Love in the Time of Cholera

Some nonfiction works are also written in narrative form. For example, some authors choose a narrative style to convey factual information about a topic, such as a specific animal, country, geographic region, and scientific or natural phenomenon.

Since narrative is the type of writing that tells a story, it must be told by someone, who is the narrator. The narrator may be a fictional character telling the story from their own viewpoint. This narrator uses the first person (*I, me, my, mine* and *we, us, our,* and *ours*). The narrator may simply be the author; for example, when Louisa May Alcott writes "Dear reader" in *Little Women*, she (the author) addresses us as readers. In this case, the novel is typically told in third person, referring to the characters as he, she, they, or them. Another more common technique is the omniscient narrator; i.e. the story is told by an unidentified individual who sees and knows everything about the events and characters—not only their externalized actions, but also their internalized feelings and thoughts. Second person, i.e. writing the story by addressing readers as "you" throughout, is less frequently used.

Expository Writing
Expository writing is also known as informational writing. Its purpose is not to tell a story as in narrative writing, to paint a picture as in descriptive writing, or to persuade readers to agree with something as in argumentative writing. Rather, its point is to communicate information to the reader. As such, the point of view of the author will necessarily be more objective. Whereas other types of writing appeal to the reader's emotions, appeal to the reader's reason by using logic, or use subjective descriptions to sway the reader's opinion or thinking, expository writing seeks to do none of these but simply to provide facts, evidence, observations, and objective descriptions of the subject matter. Some examples of expository writing include research reports, journal articles, articles and books about historical events or periods, academic subject textbooks, news articles and other factual journalistic reports, essays, how-to articles, and user instruction manuals.

Technical Writing
Technical writing is similar to expository writing in that it is factual, objective, and intended to provide information to the reader. Indeed, it may even be considered a subcategory of expository writing. However, technical writing differs from expository writing in that (1) it is specific to a particular field, discipline, or subject; and (2) it uses the specific technical terminology that belongs only to that area. Writing that uses technical terms is intended only for an audience familiar with those terms. A primary example of technical writing today is writing related to computer programming and use.

Persuasive Writing
Persuasive writing is intended to persuade the reader to agree with the author's position. It is also known as argumentative writing. Some writers may be responding to other writers' arguments, in which case they make reference to those authors or text and then disagree with them. However, another common technique is for the author to anticipate opposing viewpoints in general, both from other authors and from the author's own readers. The author brings up these opposing viewpoints, and then refutes them before they can even be raised, strengthening the author's argument. Writers persuade readers by appealing to their reason, which Aristotle called **logos;** appealing to emotion, which Aristotle called **pathos;** or appealing to readers based on the author's character and credibility, which Aristotle called **ethos.**

Evaluating the Author's Point of View in a Given Text

When a writer tells a story using the first person, readers can identify this by the use of first-person pronouns, like *I, me, we, us,* etc. However, first-person narratives can be told by different people or from different points of view. For example, some authors write in the first person to tell the story from the main character's viewpoint, as Charles Dickens did in his novels *David Copperfield* and *Great Expectations.* Some authors write in the first person from the viewpoint of a fictional character in the story, but not necessarily the main character. For example, F. Scott Fitzgerald wrote *The Great Gatsby* as narrated by Nick Carraway, a character in the story, about the main characters, Jay Gatsby and Daisy Buchanan. Other authors write in the first person, but as the omniscient narrator—an often unnamed person who knows all of the characters' inner thoughts and feelings. Writing in first person as oneself is more common in nonfiction.

Third Person

The third-person narrative is probably the most prevalent voice used in fictional literature. While some authors tell stories from the point of view and in the voice of a fictional character using the first person, it is a more common practice to describe the actions, thoughts, and feelings of fictional characters in the third person using *he, him, she, her, they, them,* etc.

Although plot and character development are both necessary and possible when writing narrative from a first-person point of view, they are also more difficult, particularly for new writers and those who find it unnatural or uncomfortable to write from that perspective. Therefore, writing experts advise beginning writers to start out writing in the third person. A big advantage of third-person narration is that the writer can describe the thoughts, feelings, and motivations of every character in a story, which is not possible for the first-person narrator. Third-person narrative can impart information to readers that the characters do not know. On the other hand, beginning writers often regard using the third-person point of view as more difficult because they must write about the feelings and thoughts of every character, rather than only about those of the protagonist.

Second Person

Narrative written in the second person addresses someone else as "you." In novels and other fictional works, the second person is the narrative voice most seldom used. The primary reason for this is that it often reads in an awkward manner, which prevents readers from being drawn into the fictional world of the novel. The second person is more often used in informational text, especially in how-to manuals, guides, and other instructions.

First Person

First person uses pronouns such as *I, me, we, my, us, and our.* Some writers naturally find it easier to tell stories from their own points of view, so writing in the first person offers advantages for them. The first-person voice is better for interpreting the world from a single viewpoint, and for enabling reader immersion in one protagonist's experiences. However, others find it difficult to use the first-person narrative voice. Its disadvantages can include overlooking the emotions of characters, forgetting to include description, producing stilted writing, using too many sentence structures involving "I did....", and not devoting enough attention to the story's "here-and-now" immediacy.

Using Text Features

Table of Contents and Index
When examining a book, a journal article, a monograph, or other publication, the table of contents is in the front. In books, it is typically found following the title page, publication information (often on the facing side of the title page), and dedication page, when one is included. In shorter publications, the table of contents may follow the title page, or the title on the same page. The table of contents in a book lists the number and title of each chapter and its beginning page number. An index, which is most common in books but may also be included in shorter works, is at the back of the publication. Books, especially academic texts, frequently have two: a subject index and an author index. Readers can look alphabetically for specific subjects in the subject index. Likewise, they can look up specific authors cited, quoted, discussed, or mentioned in the author index.

The index in a book offers particular advantages to students. For example, college course instructors typically assign certain textbooks, but do not expect students to read the entire book from cover to cover immediately. They usually assign specific chapters to read in preparation for specific lectures and/or discussions in certain upcoming classes. Reading portions at a time, some students may find references they either do not fully understand or want to know more about. They can look these topics up in the book's subject index to find them in later chapters. When a text author refers to another author, students can also look up the name in the book's author index to find all page numbers of all other references to that author. College students also typically are assigned research papers to write. A book's subject and author indexes can guide students to pages that may help inform them of other books to use for researching paper topics.

Headings
Headings and subheadings concisely inform readers what each section of a paper contains, as well as showing how its information is organized both visually and verbally. Headings are typically up to about five words long. They are not meant to give in-depth analytical information about the topic of their section, but rather an idea of its subject matter. Text authors should maintain consistent style across all headings. Readers should not expect headings if there is not material for more than one heading at each level, just as a list is unnecessary for a single item. Subheadings may be a bit longer than headings because they expand upon them. Readers should skim the subheadings in a paper to use them as a map of how content is arranged. Subheadings are in smaller fonts than headings to mirror relative importance. Subheadings are not necessary for every paragraph. They should enhance content, not substitute for topic sentences.

When a heading is brief, simple, and written in the form of a question, it can have the effect of further drawing readers into the text. An effective author will also answer the question in the heading soon in the following text. Question headings and their text answers are particularly helpful for engaging readers with average reading skills. Both headings and subheadings are most effective with more readers when they are obvious, simple, and get to their points immediately. Simple headings attract readers; simple subheadings allow readers a break, during which they also inform reader decisions whether to continue reading or not. Headings stand out from other text through boldface, but also italicizing and underlining them would be excessive. Uppercase-lowercase headings are easier for readers to comprehend than all capitals. More legible fonts are better. Some experts prefer serif fonts in text, but sans-serif fonts in headings. Brief subheadings that preview upcoming chunks of information reach more readers.

Text Features

Textbooks that are designed well employ varied text features for organizing their main ideas, illustrating central concepts, spotlighting significant details, and signaling evidence that supports the ideas and points conveyed. When a textbook uses these features in recurrent patterns that are predictable, it makes it easier for readers to locate information and come up with connections. When readers comprehend how to make use of text features, they will take less time and effort deciphering how the text is organized, leaving them more time and energy for focusing on the actual content in the text. Instructional activities can include not only previewing text through observing main text features, but moreover through examining and deconstructing the text and ascertaining how the text features can aid them in locating and applying text information for learning.

Included among various text features are a table of contents, headings, subheadings, an index, a glossary, a foreword, a preface, paragraphing spaces, bullet lists, footnotes, sidebars, diagrams, graphs, charts, pictures, illustrations, captions, italics, boldface, colors, and symbols. A **glossary** is a list of key vocabulary words and/or technical terminology and definitions. This helps readers recognize or learn specialized terms used in the text before reading it. A **foreword** is typically written by someone other than the text author and appears at the beginning to introduce, inform, recommend, and/or praise the work. A **preface** is often written by the author and also appears at the beginning, to introduce or explain something about the text, like new additions. A **sidebar** is a box with text and sometimes graphics at the left or right side of a page, typically focusing on a more specific issue, example, or aspect of the subject. **Footnotes** are additional comments/notes at the bottom of the page, signaled by superscript numbers in the text.

Text Features on Websites

On the Internet or in computer software programs, text features include URLs, home pages, pop-up menus, drop-down menus, bookmarks, buttons, links, navigation bars, text boxes, arrows, symbols, colors, graphics, logos, and abbreviations. URLs (Universal Resource Locators) indicate the internet "address" or location of a website or web page. They often start with www. (world wide web) or http:// (hypertext transfer protocol) or https:// (the "s" indicates a secure site) and appear in the Internet browser's top address bar. Clickable buttons are often links to specific pages on a website or other external sites. Users can click on some buttons to open pop-up or drop-down menus, which offer a list of actions or departments from which to select. Bookmarks are the electronic versions of physical bookmarks. When users bookmark a website/page, a link is established to the site URL and saved, enabling returning to the site in the future without having to remember its name or URL by clicking the bookmark.

Readers can more easily navigate websites and read their information by observing and utilizing their various text features. For example, most fully developed websites include search bars, where users can type in topics, questions, titles, or names to locate specific information within the large amounts stored on many sites. Navigation bars (software developers frequently use the abbreviation term "navbar") are graphical user interfaces (GUIs) that facilitate visiting different sections, departments, or pages within a website, which can be difficult or impossible to find without these. Typically, they appear as a series of links running horizontally across the top of each page. Navigation bars displayed vertically along the left side of the page are also called sidebars. Links, i.e. hyperlinks, enable hyperspeed browsing by allowing readers to jump to new pages/sites. They may be URLs, words, phrases, images, buttons, etc. They are often but not always underlined and/or blue, or other colors.

Integration of Knowledge and Ideas

Identifying Primary Sources in Various Media

A **primary source** is a piece of original work. This can include books, musical compositions, recordings, movies, works of visual art (paintings, drawings, photographs), jewelry, pottery, clothing, furniture, and other artifacts. Within books, primary sources may be of any genre. Whether nonfiction based on actual events or a fictional creation, the primary source relates the author's firsthand view of some specific event, phenomenon, character, place, process, ideas, field of study or discipline, or other subject matter. Whereas primary sources are original treatments of their subjects, secondary sources are a step removed from the original subjects; they analyze and interpret primary sources. These include journal articles, newspaper or magazine articles, works of literary criticism, political commentaries, and academic textbooks.

In the field of history, primary sources frequently include documents that were created around the same time period that they were describing, and most often produced by someone who had direct experience or knowledge of the subject matter. In contrast, secondary sources present the ideas and viewpoints of other authors about the primary sources; in history, for example, these can include books and other written works about the particular historical periods or eras in which the primary sources were produced. Primary sources pertinent in history include diaries, letters, statistics, government information, and original journal articles and books. In literature, a primary source might be a literary novel, a poem or book of poems, or a play. Secondary sources addressing primary sources may be criticism, dissertations, theses, and journal articles. Tertiary sources, typically reference works referring to primary and secondary sources, include encyclopedias, bibliographies, handbooks, abstracts, and periodical indexes.

In scientific fields, when scientists conduct laboratory experiments to answer specific research questions and test hypotheses, lab reports and reports of research results constitute examples of primary sources. When researchers produce statistics to support or refute hypotheses, those statistics are primary sources. When a scientist is studying some subject longitudinally or conducting a case study, they may keep a journal or diary. For example, Charles Darwin kept diaries of extensive notes on his studies during sea voyages on the *Beagle*, visits to the Galápagos Islands, etc.; Jean Piaget kept journals of observational notes for case studies of children's learning behaviors. Many scientists, particularly in past centuries, shared and discussed discoveries, questions, and ideas with colleagues through letters, which also constitute primary sources. When a scientist seeks to replicate another's experiment, the reported results, analysis, and commentary on the original work is a secondary source, as is a student's dissertation if it analyzes or discusses others' work rather than reporting original research or ideas.

Making Predictions and Inferences

One technique authors often use to make their fictional stories more interesting is not giving away too much information by providing hints and description. It is then up to the reader to draw a conclusion about the author's meaning by connecting textual clues with the reader's own pre-existing experiences and knowledge. Drawing conclusions is important as a reading strategy for understanding what is occurring in a text. Rather than directly stating who, what, where, when, or why, authors often describe story elements. Then, readers must draw conclusions to understand significant story components. As they go through a text, readers can think about the setting, characters, plot, problem, and solution; whether the author provided any clues for consideration; and combine any story clues with their existing knowledge and experiences to draw conclusions about what occurs in the text.

Making Predictions

Before and during reading, readers can apply the reading strategy of making predictions about what they think may happen next. For example, what plot and character developments will occur in fiction? What points will the author discuss in nonfiction? Making predictions about portions of text they have not yet read prepares readers mentally for reading, and also gives them a purpose for reading. To inform and make predictions about text, the reader can do the following:

- Consider the title of the text and what it implies
- Look at the cover of the book
- Look at any illustrations or diagrams for additional visual information
- Analyze the structure of the text
- Apply outside experience and knowledge to the text

Readers may adjust their predictions as they read. Reader predictions may or may not come true in text.

Making Inferences

Authors describe settings, characters, character emotions, and events. Readers must infer to understand text fully. Inferring enables readers to figure out meanings of unfamiliar words, make predictions about upcoming text, draw conclusions, and reflect on reading. Readers can infer about text before, during, and after reading. In everyday life, we use sensory information to infer. Readers can do the same with text. When authors do not answer all reader questions, readers must infer by saying "I think....This could be....This is because....Maybe....This means....I guess..." etc. Looking at illustrations, considering characters' behaviors, and asking questions during reading facilitate inference. Taking clues from text and connecting text to prior knowledge help to draw conclusions. Readers can infer word meanings, settings, reasons for occurrences, character emotions, pronoun referents, author messages, and answers to questions unstated in text. To practice inference, students can read sentences written/selected by the instructor, discuss the setting and character, draw conclusions, and make predictions.

Making inferences and drawing conclusions involve skills that are quite similar: both require readers to fill in information the author has omitted. Authors may omit information as a technique for inducing readers to discover the outcomes themselves; or they may consider certain information unimportant; or they may assume their reading audience already knows certain information. To make an inference or draw a conclusion about text, readers should observe all facts and arguments the author has presented and consider what they already know from their own personal experiences. Reading students taking multiple-choice tests that refer to text passages can determine correct and incorrect choices based on the information in the passage. For example, from a text passage describing an individual's signs of anxiety while unloading groceries and nervously clutching their wallet at a grocery store checkout, readers can infer or conclude that the individual may not have enough money to pay for everything.

Comparing and Contrasting Themes from Print and Other Sources

The **theme** of a piece of text is the central idea the author communicates. Whereas the topic of a passage of text may be concrete in nature, the theme is always conceptual. For example, while the topic of Mark Twain's novel *The Adventures of Huckleberry Finn* might be described as something like the coming-of-age experiences of a poor, illiterate, functionally orphaned boy around and on the Mississippi River in 19th-century Missouri, one theme of the book might be that human beings are corrupted by society. Another might be that slavery and "civilized" society itself are hypocritical. Whereas the main idea in a text is the most important single point that the author wants to make, the theme is the concept or view around which the author centers the text.

Throughout time, humans have told stories with similar themes. Some themes are universal across time, space, and culture. These include themes of the individual as a hero, conflicts of the individual against nature, the individual against society, change vs. tradition, the circle of life, coming-of-age, and the complexities of love. Themes involving war and peace have featured prominently in diverse works, like Homer's *Iliad*, Tolstoy's *War and Peace* (1869), Stephen Crane's *The Red Badge of Courage* (1895), Hemingway's *A Farewell to Arms* (1929), and Margaret Mitchell's *Gone with the Wind* (1936). Another universal literary theme is that of the quest. These appear in folklore from countries and cultures worldwide, including the Gilgamesh Epic, Arthurian legend's Holy Grail quest, Virgil's *Aeneid*, Homer's *Odyssey*, and the *Argonautica*. Cervantes' *Don Quixote* is a parody of chivalric quests. J.R.R. Tolkien's *The Lord of the Rings* trilogy (1954) also features a quest.

One instance of similar themes across cultures is when those cultures are in countries that are geographically close to each other. For example, a folklore story of a rabbit in the moon using a mortar and pestle is shared among China, Japan, Korea, and Thailand—making medicine in China, making rice cakes in Japan and Korea, and hulling rice in Thailand. Another instance is when cultures are more distant geographically, but their languages are related. For example, East Turkestan's Uighurs and people in Turkey share tales of folk hero Effendi Nasreddin Hodja. Another instance, which may either be called cultural diffusion or simply reflect commonalities in the human imagination, involves shared themes among geographically and linguistically different cultures: both Cameroon's and Greece's folklore tell of centaurs; Cameroon, India, Malaysia, Thailand, and Japan, of mermaids; Brazil, Peru, China, Japan, Malaysia, Indonesia, and Cameroon, of underwater civilizations; and China, Japan, Thailand, Vietnam, Malaysia, Brazil, and Peru, of shape-shifters.

Two prevalent literary themes are love and friendship, which can end happily, sadly, or both. William Shakespeare's *Romeo and Juliet*, Emily Brontë's *Wuthering Heights*, Leo Tolstoy's *Anna Karenina*, and both *Pride and Prejudice* and *Sense and Sensibility* by Jane Austen are famous examples. Another theme recurring in popular literature is of revenge, an old theme in dramatic literature, e.g. Elizabethans Thomas Kyd's *The Spanish Tragedy* and Thomas Middleton's *The Revenger's Tragedy*. Some more well-known instances include Shakespeare's tragedies *Hamlet* and *Macbeth*, Alexandre Dumas' *The Count of Monte Cristo*, John Grisham's *A Time to Kill*, and Stieg Larsson's *The Girl Who Kicked the Hornet's Nest*.

Themes are underlying meanings in literature. For example, if a story's main idea is a character succeeding against all odds, the theme is overcoming obstacles. If a story's main idea is one character wanting what another character has, the theme is jealousy. If a story's main idea is a character doing something they were afraid to do, the theme is courage. Themes differ from topics in that a topic is a subject matter; a theme is the author's opinion about it. For example, a work could have a topic of war and a theme that war is a curse. Authors present themes through characters' feelings, thoughts, experiences, dialogue, plot actions, and events. Themes function as "glue" holding other essential story elements together. They offer readers insights into characters' experiences, the author's philosophy, and how the world works.

Evaluating an Argument and its Specific Claims

When authors write text for the purpose of persuading others to agree with them, they assume a position with the subject matter about which they are writing. Rather than presenting information objectively, the author treats the subject matter subjectively so that the information presented supports his or her position. In their argumentation, the author presents information that refutes or weakens opposing positions. Another technique authors use in persuasive writing is to anticipate arguments against the position. When students learn to read subjectively, they gain experience with the concept of persuasion in writing, and learn to identify positions taken by authors. This enhances their reading comprehension and develops their skills for identifying pro and con arguments and biases.

There are five main parts of the classical argument that writers employ in a well-designed stance:

- Introduction: In the introduction to a classical argument, the author establishes goodwill and rapport with the reading audience, warms up the readers, and states the thesis or general theme of the argument.

- Narration: In the narration portion, the author gives a summary of pertinent background information, informs the readers of anything they need to know regarding the circumstances and environment surrounding and/or stimulating the argument, and establishes what is at risk or the stakes in the issue or topic. Literature reviews are common examples of narrations in academic writing.

- Confirmation: The confirmation states all claims supporting the thesis and furnishes evidence for each claim, arranging this material in logical order—e.g. from most obvious to most subtle or strongest to weakest.

- Refutation and Concession: The refutation and concession discuss opposing views and anticipate reader objections without weakening the thesis, yet permitting as many oppositions as possible.

- Summation: The summation strengthens the argument while summarizing it, supplying a strong conclusion and showing readers the superiority of the author's solution.

Introduction

A classical argument's introduction must pique reader interest, get readers to perceive the author as a writer, and establish the author's position. Shocking statistics, new ways of restating issues, or quotations or anecdotes focusing the text can pique reader interest. Personal statements, parallel instances, or analogies can also begin introductions—so can bold thesis statements if the author believes readers will agree. Word choice is also important for establishing author image with readers.

The introduction should typically narrow down to a clear, sound thesis statement. If readers cannot locate one sentence in the introduction explicitly stating the writer's position or the point they support, the writer probably has not refined the introduction sufficiently.

Narration and Confirmation

The narration part of a classical argument should create a context for the argument by explaining the issue to which the argument is responding, and by supplying any background information that influences the issue. Readers should understand the issues, alternatives, and stakes in the argument by the end of the narration to enable them to evaluate the author's claims equitably. The confirmation part of the classical argument enables the author to explain why they believe in the argument's thesis. The author builds a chain of reasoning by developing several individual supporting claims and explaining why that evidence supports each claim and also supports the overall thesis of the argument.

Refutation and Concession and Summation

The classical argument is the model for argumentative/persuasive writing, so authors often use it to establish, promote, and defend their positions. In the refutation aspect of the refutation and concession part of the argument, authors disarm reader opposition by anticipating and answering their possible objections, persuading them to accept the author's viewpoint. In the concession aspect, authors can concede those opposing viewpoints with which they agree. This can avoid weakening the author's thesis while establishing reader respect and goodwill for the author: all refutation and no concession can antagonize readers who disagree with the author's position. In the conclusion part of the classical argument, a less skilled writer might simply summarize or restate the thesis and related claims; however, this does not provide the argument with either momentum or closure. More skilled authors revisit the issues and the narration part of the argument, reminding readers of what is at stake.

Integrating Data from Multiple Sources in Various Formats, Including Media

Books as Resources

When a student has an assignment to research and write a paper, one of the first steps after determining the topic is to select research sources. The student may begin by conducting an Internet or library search of the topic, may refer to a reading list provided by the instructor, or may use an annotated bibliography of works related to the topic. To evaluate the worth of the book for the research paper, the student first considers the book title to get an idea of its content. Then the student can scan the book's table of contents for chapter titles and topics to get further ideas of their applicability to the topic. The student may also turn to the end of the book to look for an alphabetized index. Most academic textbooks and scholarly works have these; students can look up key topic terms to see how many are included and how many pages are devoted to them.

Journal Articles

Like books, journal articles are primary or secondary sources the student may need to use for researching any topic. To assess whether a journal article will be a useful source for a particular paper topic, a student can first get some idea about the content of the article by reading its title and subtitle, if any exists. Many journal articles, particularly scientific ones, include abstracts. These are brief summaries of the content. The student should read the abstract to get a more specific idea of whether the experiment, literature review, or other work documented is applicable to the paper topic. Students should also check the references at the end of the article, which today often contain links to related works for exploring the topic further.

Encyclopedias and Dictionaries

Dictionaries and encyclopedias are both reference books for looking up information alphabetically. Dictionaries are more exclusively focused on vocabulary words. They include each word's correct spelling, pronunciation, variants, part(s) of speech, definitions of one or more meanings, and examples used in a sentence. Some dictionaries provide illustrations of certain words when these inform the meaning. Some dictionaries also offer synonyms, antonyms, and related words under a word's entry. Encyclopedias, like dictionaries, often provide word pronunciations and definitions. However, they have broader scopes: one can look up entire subjects in encyclopedias, not just words, and find comprehensive, detailed information about historical events, famous people, countries, disciplines of study, and many other things. Dictionaries are for finding word meanings, pronunciations, and spellings; encyclopedias are for finding breadth and depth of information on a variety of topics.

Card Catalogs

A card catalog is a means of organizing, classifying, and locating the large numbers of books found in libraries. Without being able to look up books in library card catalogs, it would be virtually impossible to find them on library shelves. Card catalogs may be on traditional paper cards filed in drawers, or electronic catalogs accessible online; some libraries combine both. Books are shelved by subject area; subjects are coded using formal classification systems—standardized sets of rules for identifying and labeling books by subject and author. These assign each book a call number: a code indicating the classification system, subject, author, and title. Call numbers also function as bookshelf "addresses" where books can be located. Most public libraries use the Dewey Decimal Classification System. Most university, college, and research libraries use the Library of Congress Classification. Nursing students will also encounter the National Institute of Health's National Library of Medicine Classification System, which major collections of health sciences publications utilize.

Databases

A database is a collection of digital information organized for easy access, updating, and management. Users can sort and search databases for information. One way of classifying databases is by content, i.e. full-text, numerical, bibliographical, or images. Another classification method used in computing is by organizational approach. The most common approach is a relational database, which is tabular and defines data so they can be accessed and reorganized in various ways. A distributed database can be reproduced or interspersed among different locations within a network. An object-oriented database is organized to be aligned with object classes and subclasses defining the data. Databases usually collect files like product inventories, catalogs, customer profiles, sales transactions, student bodies, and resources. An associated set of application programs is a database management system or database manager. It enables users to specify which reports to generate, control access to reading and writing data, and analyze database usage. Structured Query Language (SQL) is a standard computer language for updating, querying, and otherwise interfacing with databases.

Practice Questions

The next two questions are based off the following passage:

Rehabilitation rather than punitive justice is becoming much more popular in prisons around the world. Prisons in America, especially, where the recidivism rate is 67 percent, would benefit from mimicking prison tactics in Norway, which has a recidivism rate of only 20 percent. In Norway, the idea is that a rehabilitated prisoner is much less likely to offend than one harshly punished. Rehabilitation includes proper treatment for substance abuse, psychotherapy, healthcare and dental care, and education programs.

1. Which of the following best captures the author's purpose?
    a. To show the audience one of the effects of criminal rehabilitation by comparison.
    b. To persuade the audience to donate to American prisons for education programs.
    c. To convince the audience of the harsh conditions of American prisons.
    d. To inform the audience of the incredibly lax system of Norway prisons.

2. Which of the following describes the word *recidivism* as it is used in the passage?
    a. The lack of violence in the prison system.
    b. The opportunity of inmates to receive therapy in prison.
    c. The event of a prisoner escaping the compound.
    d. The likelihood of a convicted criminal to reoffend.

Nutrition Facts

8 servings per container

Serving size 2/3 cup (55g)

Amount per 2/3 cup
Calories 230

% DV*		
12%	**Total Fat** 8g	
5%	Saturated Fat 1g	
	Trans Fat 0g	
0%	**Cholesterol** 0mg	
7%	**Sodium** 160mg	
12%	**Total Carbs** 37g	
14%	Dietary Fiber 4g	
	Sugars 1g	
	Added Sugars 0g	
	Protein 3g	
10%	Vitamin D 2mcg	
20%	Calcium 260mg	
45%	Iron 8mg	
5%	Potassium 235mg	

* Footnote on Daily Values (DV) and calories reference to be inserted here.

3. A customer who eats two servings of the above food would consume how many carbohydrates?
    a. 74mg
    b. 74g
    c. 460g
    d. 8g

The next three questions are based off the following passage from Virginia Woolf's Mrs. Dalloway:

> What a lark! What a plunge! For so it had always seemed to her, when, with a little squeak of the hinges, which she could hear now, she had burst open the French windows and plunged at Bourton into the open air. How fresh, how calm, stiller than this of course, the air was in the early morning; like the flap of a wave; the kiss of a wave; chill and sharp and yet (for a girl of eighteen as she then was) solemn, feeling as she did, standing there at the open window, that something awful was about to happen; looking at the flowers, at the trees with the smoke winding off them and the rooks rising, falling; standing and looking until Peter Walsh said, "Musing among the vegetables?"— was that it? —"I prefer men to cauliflowers"— was that it? He must have said it at breakfast one morning when she had gone out on to the terrace — Peter Walsh. He would be back from India one of these days, June or July, she forgot which, for his letters were awfully dull; it was his sayings one remembered; his eyes, his pocket-knife, his smile, his grumpiness and, when millions of things had utterly vanished — how strange it was! — a few sayings like this about cabbages.

4. The passage is reflective of which of the following types of writing?
    a. Persuasive
    b. Expository
    c. Technical
    d. Narrative

5. What was the narrator feeling right before Peter Walsh's voice distracted her?
    a. A spark of excitement for the morning.
    b. Anger at the larks.
    c. A sense of foreboding.
    d. Confusion at the weather.

6. What is the main point of the passage?
    a. To present the events leading up to a party.
    b. To show the audience that the narrator is resentful towards Peter.
    c. To introduce Peter Walsh back into the narrator's memory.
    d. To reveal what mornings are like in the narrator's life.

7. According to the map, which of the following is the highest points on the island?
   a. Volcano Terevaka
   b. Maunga Ana Marama
   c. Puakatike Volcano
   d. Vaka Kipo

The next question is based on the following passage from The Federalist No. 78 *by Alexander Hamilton.*

> According to the plan of the convention, all judges who may be appointed by the United States are to hold their offices *during good behavior*, which is conformable to the most approved of the State constitutions and among the rest, to that of this State. Its propriety having been drawn into question by the adversaries of that plan, is no light symptom of the rage for objection, which disorders their imaginations and judgments. The standard of good behavior for the continuance in office of the judicial magistracy, is certainly one of the most valuable of the modern improvements in the practice of government. In a monarchy it is an excellent barrier to the despotism of the prince; in a republic it is a no less excellent barrier to the encroachments and oppressions of the representative body. And it is the best expedient which can be devised in any government, to secure a steady, upright, and impartial administration of the laws.

8. What is Hamilton's point in this excerpt?
    a. To show the audience that despotism within a monarchy is no longer the standard practice in the states.
    b. To convince the audience that judges holding their positions based on good behavior is a practical way to avoid corruption.
    c. To persuade the audience that having good behavior should be the primary characteristic of a person in a government body and their voting habits should reflect this.
    d. To convey the position that judges who serve for a lifetime will not be perfect and therefore we must forgive them for their bad behavior when it arises.

9. Which of the following is an acceptable heading to insert into the blank space?

Chapter 5: Literature and Language Usage
        I. Figurative Speech
                1. Alliteration
                2. Metaphors
                3. Onomatopoeia
                4. _____
    a. Nouns
    b. Agreement
    c. Personification
    d. Syntax

10. Based on the image above, which element is under Group V, Period 6?

    a. Pb
    b. Bi
    c. Uup
    d. At

11. Felicia knew she had to be <u>prudent</u> if she was going to cross the bridge over the choppy water; one wrong move and she would be falling toward the rocky rapids.

Which of the following is the definition of the underlined word based on the context of the sentence above?

    a. Patient
    b. Afraid
    c. Dangerous
    d. Careful

The next three questions are based on the passage from Many Marriages *by Sherwood Anderson.*

There was a man named Webster lived in a town of twenty-five thousand people in the state of Wisconsin. He had a wife named Mary and a daughter named Jane and he was himself a fairly prosperous manufacturer of washing machines. When the thing happened of which I am about to write he was thirty-seven or thirty-eight years old and his one child, the daughter, was seventeen. Of the details of his life up to the time a certain revolution happened within him it will be unnecessary to speak. He was however a rather quiet man inclined to have dreams which he tried to crush out of himself in order that he function as a washing machine manufacturer; and no doubt, at odd moments, when he was on a train going some place or perhaps on Sunday afternoons in the summer when he went alone to the deserted office of the factory and sat several hours looking out at a window and along a railroad track, he gave way to dreams.

12. What does the author mean by the following sentence?

"Of the details of his life up to the time a certain revolution happened within him it will be unnecessary to speak."

    a. The details of his external life don't matter; only the details of his internal life matter.
    b. Whatever happened in his life before he had a certain internal change is irrelevant.
    c. He had a traumatic experience earlier in his life which rendered it impossible for him to speak.
    d. Before the revolution, he was a lighthearted man who always wished to speak to others no matter who they were.

13. What Point Of View is this narrative told in?
    a. First person limited
    b. First person omniscient
    c. Second person
    d. Third person

14. What did Webster do for a living?
    a. Washing machine manufacturer
    b. Train operator
    c. Leader of the revolution
    d. Stay-at-home husband

15. According to the image above, what is the temperature in Fahrenheit?
   a. 17°
   b. 20°
   c. 55°
   d. 62°

16. After Sheila recently had a coronary artery bypass, her doctor encouraged her to switch to a plant-based diet to avoid foods loaded with cholesterol and saturated fats. Sheila's doctor has given her a list of foods she can purchase in order to begin making healthy dinners, which excludes dairy (cheese, yogurt, cream), eggs, and meat. The doctor's list includes the following: pasta, marinara sauce, tofu, rice, black beans, tortilla chips, guacamole, corn, salsa, rice noodles, stir-fry vegetables, teriyaki sauce, quinoa, potatoes, yams, bananas, eggplant, pizza crust, cashew cheese, almond milk, bell pepper, and tempeh.

Which of the following dishes can Sheila make that will be okay for her to eat?

   a. Eggplant parmesan with a salad
   b. Veggie pasta with marinara sauce
   c. Egg omelet with no cheese and bell peppers
   d. Quinoa burger with cheese and French fries.

17. Maritza wanted to go to the park to swim with her friends, but when she got home, she realized that nobody was there to take her.

Follow the numbered instructions to transform the sentence above into a new sentence.
    1. Replace the phrase "wanted to go" with "went."
    2. Replace the word "but" with the word "and."
    3. Replace the word "home" with "there."
    4. Replace the phrase "nobody was there" with "they had thrown."
    5. Take out the phrase "to take."
    6. Add the words "a surprise party!" at the end of the sentence.

    a. Maritza went to the park to swim with her friends, and when she got home, she realized they had thrown her a surprise party!
    b. Maritza wanted to go to the park to swim with her friends, but when she got home, she realized they had thrown her a surprise party!
    c. Maritza went to the park to swim with her friends, and when she got there, she realized that they had thrown her a surprise party!
    d. Maritza went to the park to swim with her friends, and when she got there, she realized that nobody had thrown her a surprise party!

Use the pie chart below to answer question 18:

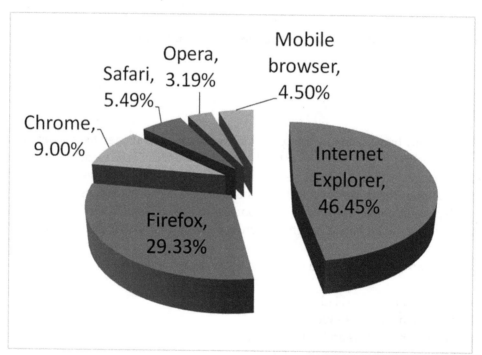

18. According to the pie chart above, which browser is most used on Wikimedia in October 2011?
    a. Firefox
    b. Chrome
    c. Safari
    d. Internet Explorer

19. A reader comes across a word they do not know in the book they are reading, and they need to find out what the word means in order to understand the context of the sentence. Where should the reader look?
   a. Table of contents
   b. Introduction
   c. Index
   d. Glossary

The next three questions are based on the following passage from the biography Queen Victoria *by E. Gordon Browne, M.A.:*

> The old castle soon proved to be too small for the family, and in September 1853 the foundation-stone of a new house was laid. After the ceremony the workmen were entertained at dinner, which was followed by Highland games and dancing in the ballroom.
>
> Two years later they entered the new castle, which the Queen described as "charming; the rooms delightful; the furniture, papers, everything perfection."
>
> The Prince was untiring in planning improvements, and in 1856 the Queen wrote: "Every year my heart becomes more fixed in this dear Paradise, and so much more so now, that *all* has become my dearest Albert's *own* creation, own work, own building, own laying out as at Osborne; and his great taste, and the impress of his dear hand, have been stamped everywhere. He was very busy today, settling and arranging many things for next year."

20. Which of the following is this excerpt considered?
   a. Primary source
   b. Secondary source
   c. Tertiary source
   d. None of these

21. How many years did it take for the new castle to be built?
   a. One year
   b. Two years
   c. Three years
   d. Four years

22. What does the word *impress* mean in the third paragraph?
   a. to affect strongly in feeling
   b. to urge something to be done
   c. to impose a certain quality upon
   d. to press a thing onto something else

Relatives Explained by Tysen

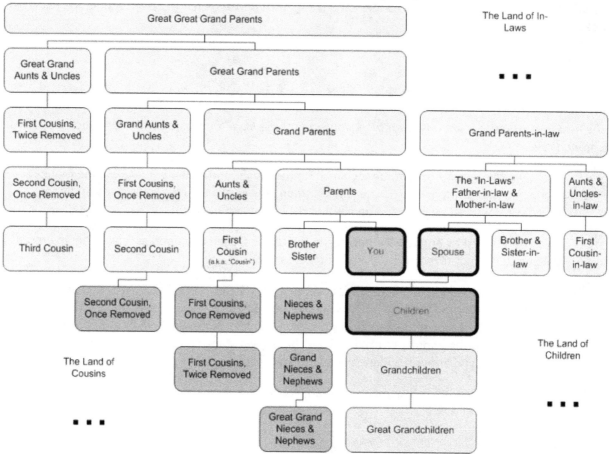

23. What does the chart mean by "Grand nieces and nephews" in relation to "You"?
    a. They are the grandchildren of your brother or sister.
    b. They are the children of your brother and sister.
    c. They are the first cousins of your brother and sister.
    d. They are the second cousins of your brother and sister.

24. What does the chart mean by "First cousin-in-law" in relation to "You"?
    a. They are the parents of your spouse.
    b. They are the aunts and uncles of your spouse.
    c. They are the cousins of your spouse.
    d. They are the children of your spouse.

The next three questions are based on the following passage from The Life, Crime, and Capture of John Wilkes Booth *by George Alfred Townsend.*

Having completed these preparations, Mr. Booth entered the theater by the stage door; summoned one of the scene shifters, Mr. John Spangler, emerged through the same door with that individual, leaving the door open, and left the mare in his hands to be held until he (Booth) should return. Booth who was even more fashionably and richly dressed than usual, walked thence around to the front of the theater, and went in. Ascending to the dress circle, he stood for a little time gazing around upon the audience and occasionally upon the stage in his usual graceful manner. He was subsequently observed by Mr. Ford, the proprietor of the theater, to be slowly elbowing his way through the crowd that packed the rear of the dress circle toward the right side, at the extremity of which was the box where Mr. and Mrs. Lincoln and their companions were seated. Mr. Ford casually noticed this as a slightly extraordinary symptom of interest on the part of an actor so familiar with the routine of the theater and the play.

25. How is the above passage organized?
   a. Chronological
   b. Cause and effect
   c. Problem to solution
   d. Main idea with supporting details

26. Based on your knowledge of history, what is about to happen?
   a. An asteroid is about to hit the earth.
   b. The best opera of all times is about to premiere.
   c. A playhouse is about to be burned to the ground.
   d. A president is about to be assassinated.

27. What does the author mean by the last two sentences?
   a. Mr. Ford was suspicious of Booth and assumed he was making his way to Mr. Lincoln's box.
   b. Mr. Ford assumed Booth's movement throughout the theater was due to being familiar with the theater.
   c. Mr. Ford thought that Booth was making his way to the theater lounge to find his companions.
   d. Mr. Ford thought that Booth was elbowing his way to the dressing room to get ready for the play.

28. A document explaining how to use an LCD flat screen TV is known as what kind of document?
   a. Technical
   b. Persuasive
   c. Narrative
   d. Cause and effect

Totok and Peranakan Population (1920 – 1971)

29. According to the graph above, what is the population of Totok in 1961?
  a. 115,000
  b. 206,000
  c. 394,000
  d. 836,000

30. According to the graph, what is the difference between the population in Peranakan in 1971 and Peranakan in 1961?
  a. 394,000
  b. 403,000
  c. 404,000
  d. 412,000

The next five questions are based on the following passage from The Story of Germ Life *by Herbert William Conn.*

When we study more carefully the effect upon the milk of the different species of bacteria found in the dairy, we find that there is a great variety of changes which they produce when they are allowed to grow in milk. The dairyman experiences many troubles with his milk. It sometimes curdles without becoming acid. Sometimes it becomes bitter, or acquires an unpleasant "tainted" taste, or, again, a "soapy" taste. Occasionally a dairyman finds his milk becoming slimy, instead of souring and curdling in the normal fashion. At such times, after a number of hours, the milk becomes so slimy that it can be drawn into long threads. Such an infection proves very troublesome, for many a time it persists in spite of all attempts made to remedy it. Again, in other cases the milk will turn blue, acquiring about the time it becomes sour a beautiful sky-blue colour. Or it may become red, or occasionally yellow. All of these troubles the dairyman owes to the presence in his milk of unusual species of bacteria which grow there abundantly.

31. What is the author's purpose in writing this passage?
    a. To show the readers that dairymen have difficult jobs.
    b. To show the readers different ways their milk might go bad.
    c. To show some of the different effects of milk on bacteria.
    d. To show some of the different effects of bacteria on milk.

32. What is the tone of this passage?
    a. Excitement
    b. Anger
    c. Neutral
    d. Sorrowful

33. Which of the following reactions does NOT occur in the above passage when bacteria infect the milk?
    a. It can have a soapy taste.
    b. The milk will turn black.
    c. It can become slimy.
    d. The milk will turn blue.

34. What is the meaning of "curdle" as depicted in the following sentence?

    Occasionally a dairyman finds his milk becoming slimy, instead of souring and <u>curdling</u> in the normal fashion.

    a. Lumpy
    b. Greasy
    c. Oily
    d. Slippery

35. Why, according to the passage, does an infection with slimy threads prove very troublesome?
    a. Because it is impossible to get rid of.
    b. Because it can make the milk-drinker sick.
    c. Because it turns the milk a blue color.
    d. Because it makes the milk taste bad.

The next question is based on the following directions.

Follow these instructions to transform the word into something new.

1. Start with the word AUDITORIUM.
2. Eliminate all vowels except for the letter O.
3. Eliminate the "T."

36. Which of the following is the new word?
    a. Door
    b. Torn
    c. Dorm
    d. Tram

37. According to the image, what's the highest speed you can measure on this odometer?
    a. 120mph
    b. 125mph
    c. 128mph
    d. 130mph

38. According to the image above, how many miles have been driven on this car?
    a. 125 miles
    b. 1,308 miles
    c. 91,308 miles
    d. 3,800 miles

39. Although Olivia felt <u>despondent</u>, she knew her sister would be home to cheer her up.

In the sentence above, what is the best definition of the underlined word?

    a. Depressed
    b. Joyful
    c. Pathetic
    d. Humorous

Portland is a very beautiful city of 60,000 inhabitants, and situated on the Willamette river twelve miles from its junction with the Columbia. It is perhaps true of many of the growing cities of the West, that they do not offer the same social advantages as the older cities of the East. But this is principally the case as to what may be called boom cities, where the larger part of the population is of that floating class which follows in the line of temporary growth for the purposes of speculation, and in no sense applies to those centers of trade whose prosperity is based on the solid foundation of legitimate business. As the metropolis of a vast section of country, having broad agricultural valleys filled with improved farms, surrounded by mountains rich in mineral wealth, and boundless forests of as fine timber as the world produces, the cause of Portland's growth and prosperity is the trade which it has as the center of collection and distribution of this great wealth of natural resources, and it has attracted, not the boomer and speculator, who find their profits in the wild excitement of the boom, but the merchant, manufacturer, and investor, who seek the surer if slower channels of legitimate business and investment. These have come from the East, most of them within the last few years. They came as seeking a better and wider field to engage in the same occupations they had followed in their Eastern homes, and bringing with them all the love of polite life which they had acquired there, have established here a new society, equaling in all respects that which they left behind. Here are as fine churches, as complete a system of schools, as fine residences, as great a love of music and art, as can be found at any city of the East of equal size.

40. What is a characteristic of a "boom city," as indicated by the passage?
    a. A city that is built on solid business foundation of mineral wealth and farming.
    b. An area of land on the west coast that quickly becomes populated by residents from the east coast.
    c. A city that, due to the hot weather and dry climate, catches fire frequently, resulting in a devastating population drop.
    d. A city whose population is made up of people who seek quick fortunes rather than building a solid business foundation.

41. According to the author, Portland is:
    a. A boom city.
    b. A city on the east coast.
    c. An industrial city.
    d. A city of legitimate business.

42. What type of passage is this?
    a. A business proposition
    b. A travel guide
    c. A journal entry
    d. A scholarly article

43. What does the word *metropolis* mean in the middle of the passage?
    a. Farm
    b. Country
    c. City
    d. Valley

The following two questions are based on the excerpt from The Golden Bough *by Sir James George Frazer.*

> The other of the minor deities at Nemi was Virbius. Legend had it that Virbius was the young Greek hero Hippolytus, chaste and fair, who learned the art of venery from the centaur Chiron, and spent all his days in the greenwood chasing wild beasts with the virgin huntress Artemis (the Greek counterpart of Diana) for his only comrade.

44. Based on a prior knowledge of literature, the reader can infer this passage is taken from which of the following?
   a. A eulogy
   b. A myth
   c. A historical document
   d. A technical document

45. What is the meaning of the word "comrade" as the last word in the passage?
   a. Friend
   b. Enemy
   c. Brother
   d. Pet

Follow the directions below.
   - 1. Drive from Florida to Georgia.
   - 2. Drive from Georgia to Texas.
   - 3. Drive from Texas to Oklahoma.
   - 4. Drive from Oklahoma to California.

46. Translate the above into general cardinal directions.

   a. Drive west, then south, then north, then west.
   b. Drive north, then west, then north, then south.
   c. Drive north, then west, then north, then west.
   d. Drive south, then west, then north, then south.

The next two questions are based on the following passage from Walden *by Henry David Thoreau.*

> When I wrote the following passages, or rather the bulk of them, I lived alone, in the woods, a mile from any neighbor, in a house which I had built myself on the shore of Walden Pond, in Concord, Massachusetts, and earned my living by the labor of my hands only. I lived there two years and two months. At present I am a sojourner in civilized life again.

47. Where in a text is this passage most likely to be found?
   a. Introduction
   b. Appendix
   c. Dedication
   d. Glossary

48. What does the word *sojourner* most likely mean at the end of the passage?
- a. Illegal immigrant
- b. Temporary resident
- c. Lifetime partner
- d. Farm crop

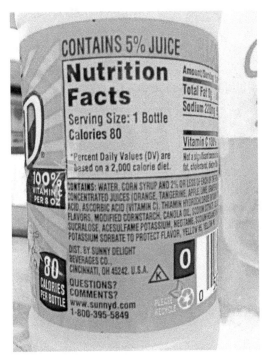

49. Based on the label above, this juice contains the most of which two ingredients?
- a. Vitamin C and cornstarch
- b. Corn syrup and Vitamin C
- c. Water and corn syrup
- d. Water and cornstarch

50. On the label above, how many calories would you consume if you drank two bottles of this drink?
- a. 80 calories
- b. 100 calories
- c. 160 calories
- d. 180 calories

The following is a preface for Poems by Alexander Pushkin *by Ivan Panin. The next three questions are based on the following passage.*

> I do not believe there are as many as five examples of deviation from the literalness of the text. Once only, I believe, have I transposed two lines for convenience of translation; the other deviations are (*if* they are such) a substitution of an *and* for a comma in order to make now and then the reading of a line musical. With these exceptions, I have sacrificed *everything* to faithfulness of rendering. My object was to make Pushkin himself, without a prompter, speak to English readers. To make him thus speak in a foreign tongue was indeed to place him at a disadvantage; and music and rhythm and harmony are indeed fine things, but truth is finer still. I wished to present not what Pushkin would have said, or [Pg 10] should have said, if he had written in English, but what he does say in Russian. That, stripped from all ornament of his

wonderful melody and grace of form, as he is in a translation, he still, even in the hard English tongue, soothes and stirs, is in itself a sign that through the individual soul of Pushkin sings that universal soul whose strains appeal forever to man, in whatever clime, under whatever sky.

51. From clues in this passage, what type of work is the author doing?
    a. Translation work
    b. Criticism
    c. Historical validity
    d. Writing a biography

52. Where would you most likely find this passage in a text?
    a. Appendix
    b. Table of contents
    c. First chapter
    d. Preface

53. According to the author, what is the most important aim of translation work?
    a. To retain the beauty of the work.
    b. To retain the truth of the work.
    c. To retain the melody of the work.
    d. To retain the form of the work.

Answer Explanations

1. A: To show the audience one of the effects of criminal rehabilitation by comparison. Choice *B* is incorrect because although it is obvious the author favors rehabilitation, the author never asks for donations from the audience. Choices *C* and *D* are also incorrect. We can infer from the passage that American prisons are probably harsher than Norway prisons. However, the best answer that captures the author's purpose is Choice *A*, because we see an effect by the author (recidivism rate of each country) comparing Norwegian and American prisons.

2. D: The likelihood of a convicted criminal to reoffend. The passage explains how a Norwegian prison, due to rehabilitation, has a smaller rate of recidivism. Thus, we can infer that recidivism is probably not a positive attribute. Choices *A* and *B* are both positive attributes, the lack of violence and the opportunity of inmates to receive therapy, so Norway would probably not have a lower rate of these two things. Choice *C* is possible, but it does not make sense in context, because the author does not talk about tactics in which to keep prisoners inside the compound, but ways in which to rehabilitate criminals so that they can live as citizens when they get out of prison.

3. B: 74g. Choice *A* has the correct number, but the unit of measurement is in "mg" instead of "g." Choices *C* and *D* are incorrect.

4. D: The passage is reflective of a narrative. A narrative is used to tell a story, as we see the narrator trying to do in this passage by using memory and dialogue. Choice *A*, persuasive writing, uses rhetorical devices to try and convince the audience of something, and there is no persuasion or argument within this passage. Choice *B*, expository, is a type of writing used to inform the reader. Choice *C*, technical writing, is usually used within business communications and uses technical language to explain procedures or concepts to someone within the same technical field.

5. C: A sense of foreboding. The narrator, after feeling excitement for the morning, feels "that something awful was about to happen," which is considered foreboding. The narrator mentions larks and weather in the passage, but there is no proof of anger or confusion at either of them.

6. C: To introduce Peter Walsh back into the narrator's memory. Choice *A* is incorrect because, although the novel *Mrs. Dalloway* is about events leading up to a party, the passage does not mention anything about a party. Choice *B* is incorrect; the narrator calls Peter *dull* at one point, but the rest of her memories of him are more positive. Choice *D* is incorrect; although morning is described within the first few sentences of the passage, the passage quickly switches to a description of Peter Walsh and the narrator's memories of him.

7. A: According to the map, Volcano Terevaka is the highest point on the island, reaching 507m. Volcano Puakatike is the next highest, reaching 307m. Vaka Kipo is the next highest reaching 216m. Finally, Maunga Ana Marama is the next highest, reaching 165m.

8. B: To convince the audience that judges holding their positions based on good behavior is a practical way to avoid corruption.

9. C: Personification. The chapter on Literature and Language Use has a subsection, "Figurative Speech." The sections located under Figurative Speech all have to do with language that uses words or phrases that are different from their literal interpretation. Personification is included in figurative speech, which means giving inanimate objects human characteristics. Nouns, agreement, and syntax all have to do with grammar and usage, and are not considered figurative language.

10. B: Bi. The element listed under Group V, Period 6 in the table is Bi. The other elements are close by, but they do not fall under this group and period.

11. D: Felicia had to be prudent, or careful, if she was going to cross the bridge over the choppy water. Choice *A*, patient, is close to the word careful. However, careful makes more sense here. Choices *B* and *C* don't make sense within the context—Felicia wasn't hoping to be *afraid* or *dangerous* while crossing over the bridge, but was hoping to be careful to avoid falling.

12. B: Whatever happened in his life before he had a certain internal change is irrelevant. Choices *A, C,* and *D* use some of the same language as the original passage, like "revolution," "speak," and "details," but they do not capture the meaning of the statement. The statement is saying the details of his previous life are not going to be talked about—that he had some kind of epiphany, and moving forward in his life is what the narrator cares about.

13. B: First-person omniscient. This is the best guess with the information we have. In the world of the passage, the narrator is first-person, because we see them use the "I," but they also know the actions and thoughts of the protagonist, a character named "Webster." First-person limited tells their own story, making Choice *A* incorrect. Choice *C* is incorrect; second person uses "you" to tell the story. Third person uses "them," "they," etc., and would not fall into use of the "I" in the narrative, making Choice *D* incorrect.

14. A: Webster is a washing machine manufacturer. This question depends on reading comprehension. We see in the second sentence that Webster "was a fairly prosperous manufacturer of washing machines," making Choice A the correct answer.

15. D: 62°. Choice *A* is the Celsius temperature, not Fahrenheit. Choices *B* and *C* are incorrect, although Choice *C* is just one degree off.

16. B: Veggie pasta with marinara sauce. Choices *A* and *D* are incorrect because they both contain cheese, and the doctor gave Sheila a list *without* dairy products. Choice *C* is incorrect because the doctor is also having Sheila stay away from eggs, and the omelet has eggs in it. Choice *B* is the best answer because it contains no meat, dairy, or eggs.

17. C: Maritza went to the park to swim with her friends, and when she got there, she realized that they had thrown her a surprise party!" Following the directions carefully will result in this sentence. All the other sentences are close, but Choices *A, B,* and *D* leave at least one of the steps out.

18. D: According to the pie chart, Internet Explorer (I.E.) is the most used browser on Wikimedia in October 2011. Following that is Firefox with 23.6% usage, Chrome with 20.6% usage, and Safari with 11.2% usage.

19. D: Glossary. A glossary is a section in a book that provides brief definitions/explanations for words that the reader may not know. Choice *A* is incorrect because a table of contents shows where each section of the book is located. Choice *B* is incorrect because the introduction is usually a chapter that introduces the book about to be read. Choice *C* is incorrect because an index is usually a list of alphabetical references at the end of a book that a reader can look up to get more information.

20. B: Secondary source. This excerpt is considered a secondary source because it actively interprets primary sources. We see direct quotes from the queen, which would be considered a primary source. But since we see those quotes being interpreted and analyzed, the excerpt becomes a secondary source. Choice *C*, tertiary source, is an index of secondary and primary sources, like an encyclopedia or Wikipedia.

21. B: It took two years for the new castle to be built. It states this in the first sentence of the second paragraph. In the third year, we see the Prince planning improvements, and arranging things for the fourth year.

22. C: To impose a certain quality upon. The sentence states that "the impress of his dear hand [has] been stamped everywhere," regarding the quality of his tastes and creations on the house. Choice *A* is one definition of *impress*, but this definition is used more as a verb than a noun: "She impressed us as a songwriter." Choice *B* is incorrect because it is also used as a verb: "He impressed the need for something to be done." Choice *D* is incorrect because it is part of a physical act: "the businessman impressed his mark upon the envelope." The phrase in the passage is meant as figurative, since the workmen did most of the physical labor, not the Prince.

23. A: They are the grandchildren of your brother and sister. Nieces and nephews refer to the children of your brother and sister, and then your grand nieces and nephews are the grandchildren of your brother and sister, and the children of your nieces and nephews.

24. C: They are the cousins of your spouse. The parents of your spouse are called your Mother-in-law or Father-in-law. The aunts and uncles of your spouse are called Aunts and Uncles-in-law. The children of your spouse would be your children or your step-children.

25. A: Chronological order. The passage presents us with a sequence of events that happens in chronological order. Choice *B* is incorrect. Cause and effect organization would usually explain why something happened or list the effects of something. Choice *C* is incorrect because problem and solution organization would detail a problem and then present a solution to the audience, and there is no solution presented here. Finally, Choice *D* is incorrect. We are entered directly into the narrative without any main idea or any kind of argument being delivered.

26. D: A president is about to be assassinated. The context clues in the passage give hints to what is about to happen. The passage mentions John Wilkes Booth as "Mr. Booth," the man who shot Abraham Lincoln. The passage also mentions a "Mr. Ford," and we know that Lincoln was shot in Ford's theater. Finally, the passage mentions Mr. and Mrs. Lincoln. By adding all these clues up and our prior knowledge of history, the assassination of President Lincoln by Booth in Ford's theater is probably the next thing that is going to happen.

27. B: Mr. Ford assumed Booth's movement throughout the theater was due to being familiar with the theater. Choice *A* is incorrect; although Booth does eventually make his way to Lincoln's box, Mr. Ford does not make this distinction in this part of the passage. Choice *C* is incorrect; although the passage mentions "companions," it mentions Lincoln's companions rather than Booth's companions. Finally, Choice *D* is incorrect; the passage mentions "dress circle," which means the first level of the theater, but this is different from a "dressing room."

28. A: Technical document. Technical documents are documents that describe the functionality of a technical product, so Choice *A* is the best answer. Persuasive texts, Choice *B*, try to persuade an audience to follow the author's line of thinking or to act on something. Choice *C*, narrative texts, seek to tell a story. Choice *D*, cause and effect, try to show why something happened, or the causes or effects of a particular thing.

29. C: 394,000. Choice *A* is the population of Totok in 1920. Choice *B* is the population of Totok in 1930. Choice *D* is the population of Peranakan in 1956 and 1961.

30. C: The answer is 404,000. This question requires some simple math by subtracting the total population of Peranakan in 1971 (1,240,000) from the total population of Peranakan in 1961 (836,000) which comes to 404,000.

31. D: To show some of the different effects of bacteria on milk. The passage explains the different ways bacteria can affect milk by detailing the color and taste of different infections. Choices *A* and *B* might be true, but they are not the main purpose of the passage as detailed in the first sentence. Choice *C* is incorrect, since milk does not have an effect on bacteria in this particular passage.

32. C: The tone of this passage is neutral, since it is written in an academic/informative voice. It is important to look at the author's word choice to determine what the tone of a passage is. We have no indication that the author is excited, angry, or sorrowful at the effects of bacteria on milk, so Choices *A, B,* and *D* are incorrect.

33. B: The milk will turn black is not a reaction mentioned in the passage. The passage does state, however, that the milk may get "soapy," that it can become "slimy," and that it may turn out to be a "beautiful sky-blue colour," making Choices *A, C,* and *D* incorrect.

34. A: Lumpy. In the sentence, we know that the word "curdle" means the opposite of "slimy." The words greasy, oily, and slippery are all very similar to the word slimy, making Choices *B, C,* and *D* incorrect. "Lumpy" means clotted, chunky, or thickened.

35. A: Because it is impossible to get rid of. The passage mentions milk turning blue or tasting bad, and milk could possibly even make a milk-drinker sick if it has slimy threads. However, we know for sure that the slimy threads prove troublesome because it can become impossible to get rid of from this sentence: "Such an infection proves very troublesome, for many a time it persists in spite of all attempts made to remedy it."

36. C: Dorm. Eliminating all vowels but the "O" makes Choice *D* incorrect. The "T" is also eliminated, which makes Choice *B* incorrect. *A* is incorrect because there is only one "O" in "auditorium."

37. B: 125mph. We see the number on the odometer reach 120mph, and then there are five marks after the 120, making the top speed 125 mph.

38. C: 91,308 miles. We can see the number of miles driven by the digital numbers underneath the odometer.

39. A: Depressed. We can guess that the word "despondent" means "depressed" by the end of the sentence. We see that although Olivia feels despondent, her sister can "cheer her up." When someone needs cheering up, they are usually sad or depressed about something. Joyful and humorous, Choices *B* and *D*, have opposite meanings of the word "despondent." Choice *C*, pathetic, is close, but Choice *A* is the best option for the context of the sentence.

40. D: A city whose population is made up of people who seek quick fortunes rather than building a solid business foundation. Choice *A* is a characteristic of Portland, but not that of a boom city. Choice *B* is close—a boom city is one that becomes quickly populated, but it is not necessarily always populated by residents from the east coast. Choice *C* is incorrect because a boom city is not one that catches fire frequently, but one made up of people who are looking to make quick fortunes from the resources provided on the land.

41. D: A city of legitimate business. We can see the proof in this sentence: "the cause of Portland's growth and prosperity is the trade which it has as the center of collection and distribution of this great wealth of natural resources, and it has attracted, not the boomer and speculator . . . but the merchant, manufacturer, and investor, who seek the surer if slower channels of legitimate business and investment." Choices *A*, *B*, and *C* are not mentioned in the passage and are incorrect.

42. B: A travel guide. Our first hint is in the title: *Oregon, Washington, and Alaska. Sights and Scenes for the Tourist*. Although the passage talks about business, there is no proposition included, which makes Choice *A* incorrect. Choice *C* is incorrect because the style of the writing is more informative and formal rather than personal and informal. Choice *D* is incorrect; this could possibly be a scholarly article, but the best choice is that it is a travel guide, due to the title and the details of what the city has to offer at the very end.

43. C: Metropolis means city. Portland is described as having agricultural valleys, but it is not solely a "farm" or "valley," making Choices *A* and *D* incorrect. We know from the description of Portland that it is more representative of a city than a countryside or country, making Choice *B* incorrect.

44. B: A myth. Look for the key words that give away the type of passage this is, such as "deities," "Greek hero," "centaur," and the names of demigods like Artemis. A eulogy is typically a speech given at a funeral, making Choice *A* incorrect. Choices *C* and *D* are incorrect, as "virgin huntresses" and "centaurs" are typically not found in historical or professional documents.

45. A: Friend. Based on the context of the passage, we can see that Hippolytus was a friend to Artemis because he "spent all his days in the greenwood chasing wild beasts" with her. The other choices are incorrect.

46. C: From Florida to Georgia is north. From Georgia to Texas is west. From Texas to Oklahoma is north. From Oklahoma to California is west.

47. A: Introduction. The passage tells us how the following passages of the book are written, which acts as an introduction to the work. An appendix comes at the end of a book, giving extra details, making Choice *B* incorrect. Choice *C* is incorrect; a dedication is at the beginning of a book, but usually acknowledges those the author is grateful towards. Choice *D* is incorrect because a glossary is a list of terms with definitions at the end of a chapter or book.

48. B: Temporary resident. Although we don't have much context to go off of, we know that one is probably not a "lifetime partner" or "farm crop" of civilized life. These two do not make sense, so Choices *C* and *D* are incorrect. Choice *A* is also a bit strange. To be an "illegal immigrant" of civilized life is not a used phrase, making Choice *A* incorrect.

49. C: Water and corn syrup. The list of ingredients on a food or drink label go from the most common ingredient found to the least common ingredient found. Water and corn syrup are both at the very top of the list. Cornstarch is found in the ingredients, but it is not at the top of the list.

50. C: 160 calories. You would consume 160 calories because one serving of this drink has 80 calories. If you double 80 calories, that gives you 160 calories. The other answer choices are incorrect.

51. A: The author is doing translation work. We see this very clearly in the way the author talks about staying truthful to the original language of the text. The text also mentions "translation" towards the end. Criticism is taking an original work and analyzing it, making Choice *B* incorrect. The work is not being tested for historical validity, but being translated into the English language, making Choice *C* incorrect. The author is not writing a biography, as there is nothing in here about Pushkin himself, only his work, making Choice *D* incorrect.

52. D: You would most likely find this in the preface. A preface to a text usually explains what the author has done or aims to do with the work. An appendix is usually found at the end of a text and does not talk about what the author intends to do to the work, making Choice *A* incorrect. A table of contents does not contain prose, but bullet points listing chapters and sections found in the text, making Choice *B* incorrect. Choice *C* is incorrect; the first chapter would include the translation work (here, poetry), and not the author's intentions.

53. B: To retain the truth of the work. The author says that "music and rhythm and harmony are indeed fine things, but truth is finer still," which means that the author stuck to a literal translation instead of changing up any words that might make the English language translation sound better.

Mathematics

Numbers and Algebra

Definitions

Whole numbers are the numbers 0, 1, 2, 3, ... Examples of other whole numbers would be 413 and 8,431. Notice that numbers such as 4.13 and $\frac{1}{4}$ are not included in whole numbers. **Counting numbers**, also known as **natural numbers**, consist of all whole numbers except for the zero. In set notation, the natural numbers are the set $\{1, 2, 3, ...\}$. The entire set of whole numbers and negative versions of those same numbers comprise the set of numbers known as **integers.** Therefore, in set notation, the integers are $\{..., -3, -2, -1, 0, 1, 2, 3, ...\}$. Examples of other integers are $-4,981$ and 90,131. A number line is a great way to visualize the integers. Integers are labeled on the following number line:

The arrows on the right- and left-hand sides of the number line show that the line continues indefinitely in both directions.

Fractions also exist on the number line as parts of a whole. For example, if an entire pie is cut into two pieces, each piece is half of the pie, or $\frac{1}{2}$. The top number in any fraction, known as the **numerator,** defines how many parts there are. The bottom number, known as the **denominator,** states how many pieces the whole is divided into. Fractions can also be negative or written in their corresponding decimal form.

A **decimal** is a number that uses a decimal point and numbers to the right of the decimal point representing the part of the number that is less than 1. For example, 3.5 is a decimal and is equivalent to the fraction $\frac{7}{2}$ or mixed number $3\frac{1}{2}$. The decimal is found by dividing 2 into 7. Other examples of fractions are $\frac{2}{7}, \frac{-3}{14}$, and $\frac{14}{27}$.

Any number that can be expressed as a fraction is known as a **rational number.** Basically, if a and b are any integers and $b \neq 0$, then $\frac{a}{b}$ is a rational number. Any integer can be written as a fraction where the denominator is 1, so therefore the rational numbers consist of all fractions and all integers.

Any number that is not rational is known as an **irrational number.** Consider the number $\pi = 3.141592654 \dots$. The decimal portion of that number extends indefinitely. In that situation, a number can never be written as a fraction. Another example of an irrational number is $\sqrt{2} = 1.414213662 \dots$ Again, this number cannot be written as a ratio of two integers.

Together, the set of all rational and irrational numbers makes up the real numbers. The number line contains all real numbers. To graph a number other than an integer on a number line, it needs to be plotted between two integers. For example, 3.5 would be plotted halfway between 3 and 4.

Even numbers are integers that are divisible by 2. For example, 6, 100, 0, and −200 are all even numbers. Odd numbers are integers that are not divisible by 2. If an odd number is divided by 2, the result is a fraction. For example, −5, 11, and −121 are odd numbers.

Prime numbers consist of natural numbers greater than 1 that are not divisible by any other natural numbers other than themselves and 1. For example, 3, 5, and 7 are prime numbers. If a natural number is not prime, it is known as a **composite number**. 8 is a composite number because it is divisible by both 2 and 4, which are natural numbers other than itself and 1.

The **absolute value** of any real number is the distance from that number to 0 on the number line. The absolute value of a number can never be negative. For example, the absolute value of both 8 and −8 is 8 because they are both 8 units away from 0 on the number line. This is written as $|8| = |-8| = 8$.

Factorization

Factorization is the process of breaking up a mathematical quantity, such as a number or polynomial, into a product of two or more factors. For example, a factorization of the number 16 is $16 = 8 \cdot 2$. If multiplied out, the factorization results in the original number. A **prime factorization** is a specific factorization when the number is factored completely using prime numbers only. For example, the prime factorization of 16 is $16 = 2 \cdot 2 \cdot 2 \cdot 2$. A factor tree can be used to find the prime factorization of any number. Within a factor tree, pairs of factors are found until no other factors can be used, as in the following factor tree of the number 84:

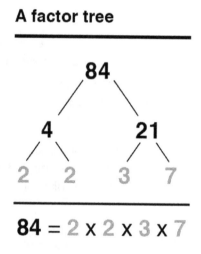

A factor tree

$$84 = 2 \times 2 \times 3 \times 7$$

It first breaks 84 into $21 \cdot 4$, which is not a prime factorization. Then, both 21 and 4 are factored into their primes. The final numbers on each branch consist of the numbers within the prime factorization. Therefore, $84 = 2 \cdot 2 \cdot 3 \cdot 7$. Factorization can be helpful in finding greatest common divisors and least common denominators.

Also, a factorization of an algebraic expression can be found. Throughout the process, a more complicated expression can be decomposed into products of simpler expressions. To factor a polynomial, first determine if there is a greatest common factor. If there is, factor it out. For example, $2x^2 + 8x$ has a greatest common factor of $2x$ and can be written as $2x(x + 4)$. Once the greatest common monomial factor is factored out, if applicable, count the number of terms in the polynomial. If there are two terms, is it a difference of squares, a sum of cubes, or a difference of cubes?

If so, the following rules can be used:

$$a^2 - b^2 = (a + b)(a - b)$$

$$a^3 + b^3 = (a + b)(a^2 - ab + b^2)$$

$$a^3 - b^3 = (a + b)(a^2 + ab + b^2)$$

If there are three terms, and if the trinomial is a perfect square trinomial, it can be factored into the following:

$$a^2 + 2ab + b^2 = (a + b)^2$$

$$a^2 - 2ab + b^2 = (a - b)^2$$

If not, try factoring into a product of two binomials by trial and error into a form of $(x + p)(x + q)$. For example, to factor $x^2 + 6x + 8$, determine what two numbers have a product of 8 and a sum of 6. Those numbers are 4 and 2, so the trinomial factors into $(x + 2)(x + 4)$.

Finally, if there are four terms, try factoring by grouping. First, group terms together that have a common monomial factor. Then, factor out the common monomial factor from the first two terms. Next, look to see if a common factor can be factored out of the second set of two terms that results in a common binomial factor. Finally, factor out the common binomial factor of each expression, for example:

$$xy - x + 5y - 5 = x(y - 1) + 5(y - 1)$$

$$(y - 1)(x + 5)$$

After the expression is completely factored, check to see if the factorization is correct by multiplying to try to obtain the original expression. Factorizations are helpful in solving equations that consist of a polynomial set equal to 0. If the product of two algebraic expressions equals 0, then at least one of the factors is equal to 0. Therefore, factor the polynomial within the equation, set each factor equal to 0, and solve. For example, $x^2 + 7x - 18 = 0$ can be solved by factoring into:

$$(x + 9)(x - 2) = 0$$

Set each factor equal to 0, and solve to obtain $x = -9$ and $x = 2$.

Converting Non-Negative Fractions, Decimals, and Percentages

Within the number system, different forms of numbers can be used. It is important to be able to recognize each type, as well as work with, and convert between, the given forms. The **real number system** comprises natural numbers, whole numbers, integers, rational numbers, and irrational numbers. Natural numbers, whole numbers, integers, and irrational numbers typically are not represented as fractions, decimals, or percentages. Rational numbers, however, can be represented as any of these three forms. A **rational number** is a number that can be written in the form $\frac{a}{b}$, where a and b are integers, and b is not equal to zero. In other words, rational numbers can be written in a fraction form. The value a is the **numerator,** and b is the **denominator.** If the numerator is equal to zero, the entire fraction is equal to zero. Non-negative fractions can be less than 1, equal to 1, or greater than 1. Fractions are less than 1 if the numerator is smaller (less than) than the denominator. For example, $\frac{3}{4}$ is less than 1. A fraction is equal to 1 if the numerator is equal to the denominator. For instance, $\frac{4}{4}$ is equal to 1. Finally, a fraction is greater than 1 if the numerator is greater than the denominator: the fraction $\frac{11}{4}$ is greater than 1. When the numerator is greater than the denominator, the fraction is called an **improper fraction**. An improper fraction can be converted to a **mixed number**, a combination of both a whole number and a fraction. To convert an improper fraction to a mixed number, divide the numerator by the denominator. Write down the whole number portion, and then write any remainder over the original denominator. For example, $\frac{11}{4}$ is equivalent to $2\frac{3}{4}$. Conversely, a mixed number can be converted to an improper fraction by multiplying the denominator times the whole number and adding that result to the numerator.

Fractions can be converted to decimals. With a calculator, a fraction is converted to a decimal by dividing the numerator by the denominator. For example:

$$\frac{2}{5} = 2 \div 5 = 0.4$$

Sometimes, rounding might be necessary. Consider:

$$\frac{2}{7} = 2 \div 7 = 0.28571429$$

This decimal could be rounded for ease of use, and if it needed to be rounded to the nearest thousandth, the result would be 0.286. If a calculator is not available, a fraction can be converted to a decimal manually. First, find a number that, when multiplied by the denominator, has a value equal to 10, 100, 1,000, etc. Then, multiply both the numerator and denominator times that number. The decimal form of the fraction is equal to the new numerator with a decimal point placed as many place values to the left as there are zeros in the denominator. For example, to convert $\frac{3}{5}$ to a decimal, multiply both the numerator and denominator times 2, which results in $\frac{6}{10}$. The decimal is equal to 0.6 because there is one zero in the denominator, and so the decimal place in the numerator is moved one unit to the left. In the case where rounding would be necessary while working without a calculator, an approximation must be found. A number close to 10, 100, 1,000, etc. can be used. For example, to convert $\frac{1}{3}$ to a decimal, the numerator and denominator can be multiplied by 33 to turn the denominator into approximately 100, which makes for an easier conversion to the equivalent decimal. This process results in $\frac{33}{99}$ and an approximate decimal of 0.33. Once in decimal form, the number can be converted to a percentage. Multiply the decimal by 100 and then place a percent sign after the number. For example, .614 is equal to 61.4%. In other words, move the decimal place two units to the right and add the percentage symbol.

Performing Arithmetic Operations with Rational Numbers

The four basic operations include addition, subtraction, multiplication, and division. The result of addition is a sum, the result of subtraction is a difference, the result of multiplication is a product, and the result of division is a quotient. Each type of operation can be used when working with rational numbers; however, the basic operations need to be understood first while using simpler numbers before working with fractions and decimals.

Performing these operations should first be learned using whole numbers. Addition needs to be done column by column. To add two whole numbers, add the ones column first, then the tens columns, then the hundreds, etc. If the sum of any column is greater than 9, a one must be carried over to the next column. For example, the following is the result of 482 + 924:

$$\begin{array}{r} 1 \\ 482 \\ +924 \\ \hline 1406 \end{array}$$

Notice that the sum of the tens column was 10, so a one was carried over to the hundreds column. Subtraction is also performed column by column. Subtraction is performed in the ones column first, then the tens, etc. If the number on top is smaller than the number below, a one must be borrowed from the column to the left. For example, the following is the result of 5,424 – 756:

$$\begin{array}{r} 4\ 13\ 11\ 14 \\ 5\ \ 4\ \ 2\ \ 4 \\ -\ 7\ \ 5\ \ 6 \\ \hline 4\ \ 6\ \ 6\ \ 8 \end{array}$$

Notice that a one is borrowed from the tens, hundreds, and thousands place. After subtraction, the answer can be checked through addition. A check of this problem would be to show that 756 + 4,668 = 5,424.

Multiplication of two whole numbers is performed by writing one on top of the other. The number on top is known as the **multiplicand,** and the number below is the **multiplier.** Perform the multiplication by multiplying the multiplicand by each digit of the multiplier. Make sure to place the ones value of each result under the multiplying digit in the multiplier. Each value to the right is then a 0. The product is found by adding each product.

For example, the following is the process of multiplying 46 times 37 where 46 is the multiplicand and 37 is the multiplier:

61

Finally, division can be performed using long division. When dividing a number by another number, the first number is known as the **dividend,** and the second is the **divisor.** For example, with $a \div b = c$, a is the dividend, b is the divisor, and c is the quotient. For long division, place the dividend within the division symbol and the divisor on the outside. For example, with $8,764 \div 4$, refer to the first problem in the diagram below. First, there are 2 4's in the first digit, 8. This number 2 gets written above the 8. Then, multiply 4 times 2 to get 8, and that product goes below the 8. Subtract to get 8, and then carry down the 7. Continue the same steps. $7 \div 4 = 1$ R3, so 1 is written above the 7. Multiply 4 times 1 to get 4, and write it below the 7. Subtract to get 3, and carry the 6 down next to the 3. Resulting steps give a 9 and a 1. The final subtraction results in a 0, which means that 8,764 is divisible by 4. There are no remaining numbers.

The second example shows that $4,536 \div 216 = 21$. The steps are a little different because 216 cannot be contained in 4 or 5, so the first step is placing a 2 above the 3 because there are 2 216's in 453. Finally, the third example shows that $546 \div 31 = 17$ R19. The 19 is a remainder. Notice that the final subtraction does not result in a 0, which means that 546 is not divisible by 31. The remainder can also be written as a fraction over the divisor to say that $546 \div 31 = 17\frac{19}{31}$.

$$
\begin{array}{r}
2191 \\
4\overline{\smash{)}8764} \\
8 \\
\hline
07 \\
4 \\
\hline
36 \\
36 \\
\hline
04 \\
4 \\
\hline
0
\end{array}
\qquad
\begin{array}{r}
21 \\
216\overline{\smash{)}4536} \\
432 \\
\hline
216 \\
216 \\
\hline
0
\end{array}
\qquad
\begin{array}{r}
17 \text{ r } 19 \\
31\overline{\smash{)}546} \\
31 \\
\hline
236 \\
217 \\
\hline
19
\end{array}
$$

If a division problem relates to a real-world application, and a remainder does exist, it can have meaning. For example, consider the third example, $546 \div 31 = 17R19$. Let's say that we had \$546 to spend on calculators that cost \$31 each, and we wanted to know how many we could buy. The division problem would answer this question. The result states that 17 calculators could be purchased, with \$19 left over. Notice that the remainder will never be greater than or equal to the divisor.

Once the operations are understood with whole numbers, they can be used with integers. There are many rules surrounding operations with negative numbers. First, consider addition with integers. The sum of two numbers can first be shown using a number line. For example, to add $-5 + (-6)$, plot the point -5 on the number line. Then, because a negative number is being added, move 6 units to the left. This process results in landing on -11 on the number line, which is the sum of -5 and -6. If adding a positive number, move to the right. Visualizing this process using a number line is useful for understanding; however, it is not efficient. A quicker process is to learn the rules. When adding two numbers with the same sign, add the absolute values of both numbers, and use the common sign of both numbers as the sign of the sum. For example, to add $-5 + (-6)$, add their absolute values $5 + 6 = 11$. Then, introduce a negative number because both addends are negative. The result is -11. To add two integers with unlike signs, subtract the lesser absolute value from the greater absolute value, and apply the sign of the number with the greater absolute value to the result. For example, the sum $-7 + 4$ can be computed by finding the difference $7 - 4 = 3$ and then applying a negative because the value with the larger absolute value is negative. The result is -3. Similarly, the sum $-4 + 7$ can be found by computing the same difference but leaving it as a positive result because the addend with the larger absolute value is positive. Also, recall that any number plus 0 equals that number. This is known as the **Addition Property of 0.**

Subtracting two integers can be computed by changing to addition to avoid confusion. The rule is to add the first number to the opposite of the second number. The opposite of a number is the number on the other side of 0 on the number line, which is the same number of units away from 0. For example, -2 and 2 are opposites. Consider $4 - 8$. Change this to adding the opposite as follows: $4 + (-8)$. Then, follow the rules of addition of integers to obtain -4. Secondly, consider $-8 - (-2)$. Change this problem to adding the opposite as $-8 + 2$, which equals -6. Notice that subtracting a negative number is really adding a positive number.

Multiplication and division of integers are actually less confusing than addition and subtraction because the rules are simpler to understand. If two factors in a multiplication problem have the same sign, the result is positive. If one factor is positive and one factor is negative, the result, known as the **product,** is negative. For example, $(-9)(-3) = 27$ and $9(-3) = -27$. Also, a number times 0 always results in 0. If a problem consists of more than a single multiplication, the result is negative if it contains an odd number of negative factors, and the result is positive if it contains an even number of negative factors. For example, $(-1)(-1)(-1)(-1) = 1$ and $(-1)(-1)(-1)(-1)(-1) = 1$. These two examples of multiplication also bring up another concept. Both are examples of repeated multiplication, which can be written in a more compact notation using exponents. The first example can be written as $(-1)^4 = 1$, and the second example can be written as $(-1)^5 = -1$. Both are exponential expressions, -1 is the base in both instances, and 4 and 5 are the respective exponents. Note that a negative number raised to an odd power is always negative, and a negative number raised to an even power is always positive. Also, $(-1)^4$ is not the same as -1^4. In the first expression, the negative is included in the parentheses, but it is not in the second expression. The second expression is found by evaluating 1^4 first to get 1 and then by applying the negative sign to obtain -1.

A similar theory applies within division. First, consider some vocabulary. When dividing 14 by 2, it can be written in the following ways: $14 \div 2 = 7$ or $\frac{14}{2} = 7$. 14 is the **dividend,** 2 is the **divisor,** and 7 is the **quotient.** If two numbers in a division problem have the same sign, the quotient is positive. If two numbers in a division problem have different signs, the quotient is negative. For example:

$$14 \div (-2) = -7, \text{ and } -14 \div (-2) = 7$$

To check division, multiply the quotient times the divisor to obtain the dividend. Also, remember that 0 divided by any number is equal to 0. However, any number divided by 0 is undefined. It just does not make sense to divide a number by 0 parts.

If more than one operation is to be completed in a problem, follow the **Order of Operations**. The mnemonic device, PEMDAS, for the order of operations states the order in which addition, subtraction, multiplication, and division need to be done. It also includes when to evaluate operations within grouping symbols and when to incorporate exponents. PEMDAS, which some remember by thinking "please excuse my dear Aunt Sally," refers to parentheses, exponents, multiplication, division, addition, and subtraction. First, within an expression, complete any operation that is within parentheses, or any other grouping symbol like brackets, braces, or absolute value symbols. Note that this does not refer to the case when parentheses are used to represent multiplication like (2)(5). An operation is not within parentheses like it is in (2 · 5). Then, any exponents must be computed. Next, multiplication and division are performed from left to right.

Finally, addition and subtraction are performed from left to right. The following is an example in which the operations within the parentheses need to be performed first, so the order of operations must be applied to the exponent, subtraction, addition, and multiplication within the grouping symbol:

$$9 - 3(3^2 - 3 + 4 \cdot 3)$$

$$9 - 3(3^2 - 3 + 4 \cdot 3)$$ \quad \text{Work within the parentheses first}

$$= 9 - 3(9 - 3 + 12)$$

$$= 9 - 3(18)$$

$$= 9 - 54$$

$$= -45$$

Once the rules for integers are understood, move on to learning how to perform operations with fractions and decimals. Recall that a rational number can be written as a fraction and can be converted to a decimal through division. If a rational number is negative, the rules for adding, subtracting, multiplying, and dividing integers must be used. If a rational number is in fraction form, performing addition, subtraction, multiplication, and division is more complicated than when working with integers. First, consider addition. To add two fractions having the same denominator, add the numerators and then reduce the fraction. When an answer is a fraction, it should always be in lowest terms. **Lowest terms** means that every common factor, other than 1, between the numerator and denominator is divided out. For example:

$$\frac{2}{8} + \frac{4}{8} = \frac{6}{8} = \frac{6 \div 2}{8 \div 2} = \frac{3}{4}$$

Both the numerator and denominator of $\frac{6}{8}$ have a common factor of 2, so 2 is divided out of each number to put the fraction in lowest terms. If denominators are different in an addition problem, the fractions must be converted to have common denominators. The **least common denominator (LCD)** of all the given denominators must be found, and this value is equal to the **least common multiple (LCM)** of the denominators. This non-zero value is the smallest number that is a multiple of both denominators. Then, rewrite each original fraction as an equivalent fraction using the new denominator. Once in this form, apply the process of adding with like denominators. For example, consider $\frac{1}{3} + \frac{4}{9}$. The LCD is 9 because it is the smallest multiple of both 3 and 9. The fraction $\frac{1}{3}$ must be rewritten with 9 as its denominator.

Therefore, multiply both the numerator and denominator times 3. Multiplying times $\frac{3}{3}$ is the same as multiplying times 1, which does not change the value of the fraction. Therefore, an equivalent fraction is $\frac{3}{9}$, and $\frac{1}{3} + \frac{4}{9} = \frac{3}{9} + \frac{4}{9} = \frac{7}{9}$, which is in lowest terms. Subtraction is performed in a similar manner; once the denominators are equal, the numerators are then subtracted. The following is an example of addition of a positive and a negative fraction:

$$-\frac{5}{12} + \frac{5}{9} = -\frac{5 \cdot 3}{12 \cdot 3} + \frac{5 \cdot 4}{9 \cdot 4}$$

$$-\frac{15}{36} + \frac{20}{36} = \frac{5}{36}$$

Common denominators are not used in multiplication and division. To multiply two fractions, multiply the numerators together and the denominators together. Then, write the result in lowest terms. For example:

$$\frac{2}{3} \times \frac{9}{4} = \frac{18}{12} = \frac{3}{2}$$

Alternatively, the fractions could be factored first to cancel out any common factors before performing the multiplication. For example:

$$\frac{2}{3} \times \frac{9}{4} = \frac{2}{3} \times \frac{3 \times 3}{2 \times 2} = \frac{3}{2}$$

This second approach is helpful when working with larger numbers, as common factors might not be obvious. Multiplication and division of fractions are related because the division of two fractions is changed into a multiplication problem. Division of a fraction is equivalent to multiplication of the *reciprocal* of the second fraction, so that second fraction must be inverted, or "flipped," to be in reciprocal form. For example:

$$\frac{11}{15} \div \frac{3}{5} = \frac{11}{15} \times \frac{5}{3} = \frac{55}{45} = \frac{11}{9}$$

The fraction $\frac{5}{3}$ is the reciprocal of $\frac{3}{5}$. It is possible to multiply and divide numbers containing a mix of integers and fractions. In this case, convert the integer to a fraction by placing it over a denominator of 1. For example, a division problem involving an integer and a fraction is:

$$3 \div \frac{1}{2} = \frac{3}{1} \times \frac{2}{1} = \frac{6}{1} = 6$$

Finally, when performing operations with rational numbers that are negative, the same rules apply as when performing operations with integers. For example, a negative fraction times a negative fraction results in a positive value, and a negative fraction subtracted from a negative fraction results in a negative value.

Operations can be performed on rational numbers in decimal form. Recall that to write a fraction as an equivalent decimal expression, divide the numerator by the denominator. For example:

$$\frac{1}{8} = 1 \div 8 = 0.125$$

With the case of decimals, it is important to keep track of place value. To add decimals, make sure the decimal places are in alignment so that the numbers are lined up with their decimal points and add vertically. If the numbers do not line up because there are extra or missing place values in one of the numbers, then zeros may be used as placeholders. For example, 0.123 + 0.23 becomes:

$$
\begin{array}{r}
0.123 \\
+\ \underline{0.230} \\
0.353
\end{array}
$$

Subtraction is done the same way. Multiplication and division are more complicated. To multiply two decimals, place one on top of the other as in a regular multiplication process and do not worry about lining up the decimal points. Then, multiply as with whole numbers, ignoring the decimals. Finally, in the solution, insert the decimal point as many places to the left as there are total decimal values in the original problem. Here is an example of a decimal multiplication:

$$
\begin{array}{rl}
0.52 & \textit{2 decimal places} \\
\underline{\times 0.2} & \textit{1 decimal place} \\
.104 & \textit{3 decimal places}
\end{array}
$$

The answer to 67 times 4 is 268, and because there are three decimal values in the problem, the decimal point is positioned three units to the left in the answer.

The decimal point plays an integral role throughout the whole problem when dividing with decimals. First, set up the problem in a long division format. If the divisor is not an integer, the decimal must be moved to the right as many units as needed to make it an integer. The decimal in the dividend must be moved to the right the same number of places to maintain equality. Then, division is completed normally. Here is an example of long division with decimals:

Long division with decimals

Because the decimal point is moved two units to the right in the divisor of 0.06 to turn it into the integer 6, it is also moved two units to the right in the dividend of 12.72 to make it 1,272. The result is 212, and remember that a division problem can always be checked by multiplying the answer times the divisor to see if the result is equal to the dividend.

Sometimes it is helpful to round answers that are in decimal form. First, find the place to which the rounding needs to be done. Then, look at the digit to the right of it. If that digit is 4 or less, the number in the place value to its left stays the same, and everything to its right becomes a 0. This process is known as **rounding down**. If that digit is 5 or higher, round up by increasing the place value to its left by 1, and every number to its right becomes a 0. If those 0's are in decimals, they can be dropped. For example, 0.145 rounded to the nearest hundredth place would be rounded up to 0.15, and 0.145 rounded to the nearest tenth place would be rounded down to 0.1.

Another operation that can be performed on rational numbers is the square root. Dealing with real numbers only, the positive square root of a number is equal to one of the two repeated positive factors of that number. For example, $\sqrt{49} = \sqrt{7 \cdot 7} = 7$. A **perfect square** is a number that has a whole number as its square root. Examples of perfect squares are 1, 4, 9, 16, 25, etc. If a number is not a perfect square, an approximation can be used with a calculator. For example, $\sqrt{67} = 8.185$, rounded to the nearest thousandth place. The square root of a fraction involving perfect squares involves breaking up the problem into the square root of the numerator separate from the square root of the denominator. For example:

$$\sqrt{\frac{16}{25}} = \frac{\sqrt{16}}{\sqrt{25}} = \frac{4}{5}$$

If the fraction does not contain perfect squares, a calculator can be used. Therefore, $\sqrt{\frac{2}{5}} = 0.632$, rounded to the nearest thousandth place. A common application of square roots involves the Pythagorean theorem. Given a right triangle, the sum of the squares of the two legs equals the square of the hypotenuse.

For example, consider the following right triangle:

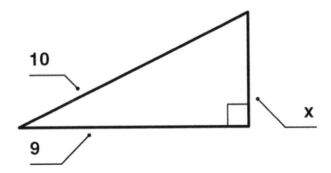

The missing side, x, can be found using the Pythagorean theorem.

$$9^2 + x^2 = 10^2$$

$$81 + x^2 = 100$$

$$x^2 = 19$$

To solve for x, take the square root of both sides. Therefore, $x = \sqrt{19} = 4.36$, which has been rounded to two decimal places.

In addition to the square root, the cube root is another operation. If a number is a **perfect cube**, the cube root of that number is equal to one of the three repeated factors. For example:

$$\sqrt[3]{27} = \sqrt[3]{3 \cdot 3 \cdot 3} = 3$$

Also, unlike square roots, a negative number has a cube root. The result is a negative number. For example:

$$\sqrt[3]{-27} = \sqrt[3]{(-3)(-3)(-3)} = -3$$

Similar to square roots, if the number is not a perfect cube, a calculator can be used to find an approximation. Therefore, $\sqrt[3]{\frac{2}{3}} = 0.873$, rounded to the nearest thousandth place.

Higher-order roots also exist. The number relating to the root is known as the **index.** Given the following root, $\sqrt[3]{64}$, 3 is the index, and 64 is the **radicand.** The entire expression is known as the **radical.** Higher-order roots exist when the index is larger than 3. They can be broken up into two groups: even and odd roots. **Even roots**, when the index is an even number, follow the properties of square roots. A negative number does not have an even root, and an even root is found by finding the single factor that is repeated the same number of times as the index in the radicand. For example, the fifth root of 32 is equal to 2 because:

$$\sqrt[5]{32} = \sqrt[5]{2 \cdot 2 \cdot 2 \cdot 2 \cdot 2} = 2$$

Odd roots, when the index is an odd number, follow the properties of cube roots. A negative number has an odd root. Similarly, an odd root is found by finding the single factor that is repeated that many times to obtain the radicand. For example, the 4th root of 81 is equal to 3 because $3^4 = 81$. This radical is written as $\sqrt[4]{81} = 4$.

When performing operations in rational numbers, sometimes it might be helpful to round the numbers in the original problem to get a rough check of what the answer should be. For example, if you walked into a grocery store and had a $20 bill, your approach might be to round each item to the nearest dollar and add up all the items to make sure that you will have enough money when you check out. This process involves obtaining an estimation of what the exact total would be. In other situations, it might be helpful to round to the nearest $10 amount or $100 amount. **Front-end rounding** might be helpful as well in many situations. In this type of rounding, each number is rounded to the highest possible place value. Therefore, all digits except the first digit become 0. Consider a situation in which you are at the furniture store and want to estimate your total on three pieces of furniture that cost $434.99, $678.99, and $129.99. Front-end rounding would round these three amounts to $400, $700, and $100. Therefore, the estimate of your total would be $400 + $700 + $100 = $1,200, compared to the exact total of $1,243.97. In this situation, the estimate is not that far off the exact answer. Rounding is useful in both approximating an answer when an exact answer is not needed and for comparison when an exact answer is needed. For instance, if you had a complicated set of operations to complete and your estimate was $1,000, if you obtained an exact answer of $100,000, something is off. You might want to check your work to see if a mistake was made because an estimate should not be that different from an exact answer. Estimates can also be helpful with square roots. If a square root of a number is not known, the closest perfect square can be found for an approximation. For example, $\sqrt{50}$ is not equal to a whole number, but 50 is close to

49, which is a perfect square, and $\sqrt{49} = 7$. Therefore, $\sqrt{50}$ is a little bit larger than 7. The actual approximation, rounded to the nearest thousandth, is 7.071.

Ordering and Comparing Rational Numbers

Ordering rational numbers is a way to compare two or more different numerical values. Determining whether two amounts are equal, less than, or greater than is the basis for comparing both positive and negative numbers. Also, a group of numbers can be compared by ordering them from the smallest amount to the largest amount. A few symbols are necessary to use when ordering rational numbers. The equals sign, =, shows that the two quantities on either side of the symbol have the same value. For example, $\frac{12}{3} = 4$ because both values are equivalent. Another symbol that is used to compare numbers is <, which represents "less than." With this symbol, the smaller number is placed on the left and the larger number is placed on the right. Always remember that the symbol's "mouth" opens up to the larger number. When comparing negative and positive numbers, it is important to remember that the number occurring to the left on the number line is always smaller and is placed to the left of the symbol. This idea might seem confusing because some values could appear at first glance to be larger, even though they are not. For example, $-5 < 4$ is read "negative 5 is less than 4." Here is an image of a number line for help:

The symbol $\leq$ represents "less than or equal to," and it joins < with equality. Therefore, both $-5 \leq 4$ and $-5 \leq -5$ are true statements and "-5 is less than or equal to both 4 and -5." Other symbols are > and $\geq$, which represent "greater than" and "greater than or equal to." Both $4 \geq -1$ and $-1 \geq -1$ are correct ways to use these symbols.

Here is a chart of these four inequality symbols:

Symbol	Definition
<	less than
$\leq$	less than or equal to
>	greater than
$\geq$	greater than or equal to

Comparing integers is a straightforward process, especially when using the number line, but the comparison of decimals and fractions is not as obvious. When comparing two non-negative decimals, compare digit by digit, starting from the left. The larger value contains the first larger digit. For example, 0.1456 is larger than 0.1234 because the value 4 in the hundredths place in the first decimal is larger than the value 2 in the hundredths place in the second decimal. When comparing a fraction with a decimal, convert the fraction to a decimal and then compare in the same manner. Finally, there are a few options when comparing fractions. If two non-negative fractions have the same denominator, the fraction with the larger numerator is the larger value. If they have different denominators, they can be converted to equivalent fractions with a common denominator to be compared, or they can be converted to decimals to be compared. When comparing two negative decimals or fractions, a different approach must be used. It is important to remember that the smaller number exists to the left on the number line. Therefore, when comparing two negative decimals by place value, the number with the larger first place value is smaller due to the negative sign. Whichever value is closer to 0 is larger. For instance, -0.456 is larger than -0.498

because of the values in the hundredth places. If two negative fractions have the same denominator, the fraction with the larger numerator is smaller because of the negative sign.

Solving Equations in One Variable

An **equation in one variable** is a mathematical statement where two algebraic expressions in one variable, usually x, are set equal. To solve the equation, the variable must be isolated on one side of the equals sign. The addition and multiplication principles of equality are used to isolate the variable. The **addition principle of equality** states that the same number can be added to or subtracted from both sides of an equation. Because the same value is being used on both sides of the equals sign, equality is maintained. For example, the equation $2x = 5x$ is equivalent to both $2x + 3 = 5x + 3$, and $2x - 5 = 5x - 5$. This principle can be used to solve the following equation: $x + 5 = 4$. The variable x must be isolated, so to move the 5 from the left side, subtract 5 from both sides of the equals sign. Therefore, $x + 5 - 5 = 4 - 5$. So, the solution is $x = -1$. This process illustrates the idea of an **additive inverse** because subtracting 5 is the same as adding -5. Basically, add the opposite of the number that must be removed to both sides of the equals sign. The **multiplication principle of equality** states that equality is maintained when a number is either multiplied times both expressions on each side of the equals sign, or when both expressions are divided by the same number. For example, $4x = 5$ is equivalent to both $16x = 20$ and $x = \frac{5}{4}$. Multiplying both sides times 4 and dividing both sides by 4 maintains equality. Solving the equation $6x - 18 = 5$ requires the use of both principles. First, apply the addition principle to add 18 to both sides of the equals sign, which results in $6x = 23$. Then use the multiplication principle to divide both sides by 6, giving the solution $x = \frac{23}{6}$. Using the multiplication principle in the solving process is the same as involving a multiplicative inverse. A **multiplicative inverse** is a value that, when multiplied by a given number, results in 1. Dividing by 6 is the same as multiplying by $\frac{1}{6}$, which is both the reciprocal and multiplicative inverse of 6.

When solving a linear equation in one variable, checking the answer shows if the solution process was performed correctly. Plug the solution into the variable in the original equation. If the result is a false statement, something was done incorrectly during the solution procedure. Checking the example above gives the following:

$$6 \times \frac{23}{6} - 18 = 23 - 18 = 5$$

Therefore, the solution is correct.

Some equations in one variable involve fractions or the use of the distributive property. In either case, the goal is to obtain only one variable term and then use the addition and multiplication principles to isolate that variable. Consider the equation $\frac{2}{3}x = 6$. To solve for x, multiply each side of the equation by the reciprocal of $\frac{2}{3}$, which is $\frac{3}{2}$. This step results in $\frac{3}{2} \times \frac{2}{3}x = \frac{3}{2} \times 6$, which simplifies into the solution $x = 9$. Now consider the equation:

$$3(x + 2) - 5x = 4x + 1$$

Use the distributive property to clear the parentheses. Therefore, multiply each term inside the parentheses by 3. This step results in:

$$3x + 6 - 5x = 4x + 1$$

Next, collect like terms on the left-hand side. **Like terms** are terms with the same variable or variables raised to the same exponent(s). Only like terms can be combined through addition or subtraction. After collecting like terms, the equation is:

$$-2x + 6 = 4x + 1$$

Finally, apply the addition and multiplication principles. Add $2x$ to both sides to obtain:

$$6 = 6x + 1$$

Then, subtract 1 from both sides to obtain $5 = 6x$. Finally, divide both sides by 6 to obtain the solution:

$$\frac{5}{6} = x$$

Two other types of solutions can be obtained when solving an equation in one variable. The final result could be that there is either no solution or that the solution set contains all real numbers. Consider the equation:

$$4x = 6x + 5 - 2x$$

First, the like terms can be combined on the right to obtain $4x = 4x + 5$. Next, subtract $4x$ from both sides. This step results in the false statement $0 = 5$. There is no value that can be plugged into x that will ever make this equation true. Therefore, there is no solution. The solution procedure contained correct steps, but the result of a false statement means that no value satisfies the equation. The symbolic way to denote that no solution exists is Ø. Next, consider the equation:

$$5x + 4 + 2x = 9 + 7x - 5$$

Combining the like terms on both sides results in:

$$7x + 4 = 7x + 4$$

The left-hand side is exactly the same as the right-hand side. Using the addition principle to move terms, the result is $0 = 0$, which is always true. Therefore, the original equation is true for any number, and the solution set is all real numbers. The symbolic way to denote such a solution set is $\mathbb{R}$, or in interval notation, $(-\infty, \infty)$.

Solving Real-World One- or Multi-Step Problems with Rational Numbers

One-step problems take only one mathematical step to solve. For example, solving the equation $5x = 45$ is a one-step problem because the one step of dividing both sides of the equation by 5 is the only step necessary to obtain the solution $x = 9$. The multiplication principle of equality is the one step used to isolate the variable. The equation is of the form $ax = b$, where a and b are rational numbers. Similarly, the addition principle of equality could be the one step needed to solve a problem. In this case, the equation would be of the form $x + a = b$ or $x - a = b$, for real numbers a and b.

A multi-step problem involves more than one step to find the solution, or it could consist of solving more than one equation. An equation that involves both the addition principle and the multiplication principle is a two-step problem, and an example of such an equation is $2x - 4 = 5$. Solving involves adding 4 to both sides and then dividing both sides by 2. An example of a two-step problem involving two separate equations is $y = 3x, 2x + y = 4$. The two equations form a system of two equations that must be solved together in two variables. The system can be solved by the substitution method. Since y is already solved for in terms of x, plug $3x$ in for y into the equation $2x + y = 4$, resulting in $2x + 3x = 4$. Therefore, $5x = 4$ and $x = \frac{4}{5}$. Because there are two variables, the solution consists of both a value for x and for y. Substitute $x = \frac{4}{5}$ into either original equation to find y. The easiest choice is $y = 3x$. Therefore:

$$y = 3 \times \frac{4}{5} = \frac{12}{5}$$

The solution can be written as the ordered pair $\left(\frac{4}{5}, \frac{12}{5}\right)$.

Real-world problems can be translated into both one-step and multi-step problems. In either case, the word problem must be translated from the verbal form into mathematical expressions and equations that can be solved using algebra. An example of a one-step real-world problem is the following: A cat weighs half as much as a dog living in the same house. If the dog weighs 14.5 pounds, how much does the cat weigh? To solve this problem, an equation can be used. In any word problem, the first step must be defining variables that represent the unknown quantities. For this problem, let x be equal to the unknown weight of the cat. Because two times the weight of the cat equals 14.5 pounds, the equation to be solved is: $2x = 14.5$. Use the multiplication principle to divide both sides by 2. Therefore, $x = 7.25$. The cat weighs 7.25 pounds.

Most of the time, real-world problems are more difficult than this one and consist of multi-step problems. The following is an example of a multi-step problem: The sum of two consecutive page numbers is equal to 437. What are those page numbers? First, define the unknown quantities. If x is equal to the first page number, then $x + 1$ is equal to the next page number because they are consecutive integers. Their sum is equal to 437, and this statement translates to the equation:

$$x + x + 1 = 437$$

To solve, first collect like terms to obtain:

$$2x + 1 = 437$$

Then, subtract 1 from both sides and then divide by 2. The solution to the equation is $x = 218$. Therefore, the two consecutive page numbers that satisfy the problem are 218 and 219. It is always important to make sure that answers to real-world problems make sense. For instance, if the solution to this same problem resulted in decimals, that should be a red flag indicating the need to check the work. Page numbers are whole numbers; therefore, if decimals are found to be answers, the solution process should be double-checked to see where mistakes were made.

Solving Real-World Problems Involving Percentages

Percentages are defined to be parts per one hundred. To convert a decimal to a percentage, move the decimal point two units to the right and place the percent sign after the number. Percentages appear in many scenarios in the real world. It is important to make sure the statement containing the percentage is translated to a correct mathematical expression. Be aware that it is extremely common to make a mistake when working with percentages within word problems.

An example of a word problem containing a percentage is the following: 35% of people speed when driving to work. In a group of 5,600 commuters, how many would be expected to speed on the way to their place of employment? The answer to this problem is found by finding 35% of 5,600. First, change the percentage to the decimal 0.35. Then compute the product: $0.35 \times 5,600 = 1,960$. Therefore, it would be expected that 1,960 of those commuters would speed on their way to work based on the data given. In this situation, the word "of" signals to use multiplication to find the answer. Another way percentages are used is in the following problem: Teachers work 8 months out of the year. What percent of the year do they work? To answer this problem, find what percent of 12 the number 8 is, because there are 12 months in a year. Therefore, divide 8 by 12, and convert that number to a percentage: $\frac{8}{12} = \frac{2}{3} = 0.66\overline{6}$. The percentage rounded to the nearest tenth place tells us that teachers work 66.7% of the year. Percentages also appear in real-world application problems involving finding missing quantities like in the following question: 60% of what number is 75? To find the missing quantity, an equation can be used. Let x be equal to the missing quantity. Therefore, $0.60x = 75$. Divide each side by 0.60 to obtain 125. Therefore, 60% of 125 is equal to 75.

Sales tax is an important application relating to percentages because tax rates are usually given as percentages. For example, a city might have an 8% sales tax rate. Therefore, when an item is purchased with that tax rate, the real cost to the customer is 1.08 times the price in the store. For example, a $25 pair of jeans costs the customer $25 \times 1.08 = $27. Sales tax rates can also be determined if they are unknown when an item is purchased. If a customer visits a store and purchases an item for $21.44, but the price in the store was $19, they can find the tax rate by first subtracting $21.44 − $19 to obtain $2.44, the sales tax amount. The sales tax is a percentage of the in-store price. Therefore, the tax rate is $\frac{2.44}{19} = 0.128$, which has been rounded to the nearest thousandths place. In this scenario, the actual sales tax rate given as a percentage is 12.8%.

Applying Estimation Strategies and Rounding Rules to Real-World Problems

Sometimes it is helpful to find an estimated answer to a problem rather than working out an exact answer. An estimation might be much quicker to find, and given the scenario, an estimation might be all that is required. For example, if Aria goes grocery shopping and has only a $100 bill to cover all of her purchases, it might be appropriate for her to estimate the total of the items she is purchasing to tell if she has enough money to cover them. Also, an estimation can help determine if an answer makes sense. For instance, if an answer in the 100s is expected, but the result is a fraction less than 1, something is probably wrong in the calculation.

The first type of estimation involves rounding. As mentioned, **rounding** consists of expressing a number in terms of the nearest decimal place like the tenth, hundredth, or thousandth place, or in terms of the nearest whole number unit like tens, hundreds, or thousands place. When rounding to a specific place value, look at the digit to the right of the place. If it is 5 or higher, round the number to its left up to the next value, and if it is 4 or lower, keep that number at the same value. For instance, 1,654.2674 rounded to the nearest thousand is 2,000, and the same number rounded to the nearest thousandth is 1,654.267. Rounding can be used in the scenario when grocery totals need to be estimated. Items can be rounded to the nearest dollar. For example, a can of corn that costs $0.79 can be rounded to $1.00, and then all other items can be rounded in a similar manner and added together.

When working with larger numbers, it might make more sense to round to higher place values. For example, when estimating the total value of a dealership's car inventory, it would make sense to round the car values to the nearest thousands place. The price of a car that is on sale for $15,654 can be estimated at $16,000. All other cars on the lot could be rounded in the same manner, and then their sum can be found. Depending on the situation, it might make sense to calculate an over-estimate. For example, to make sure Aria has enough money at the grocery store, rounding up every time for each item would ensure that she will have enough money when it comes time to pay. A $.40 item rounded up to $1.00 would ensure that there is a dollar to cover that item. Traditional rounding rules would round $0.40 to $0, which does not make sense in this particular real-world setting. Aria might not have a dollar available at checkout to pay for that item if she uses traditional rounding. It is up to the customer to decide the best approach when estimating.

Estimating is also very helpful when working with measurements. Bryan is updating his kitchen and wants to retile the floor. Again, an over-measurement might be useful. Also, rounding to nearest half-unit might be helpful. For instance, one side of the kitchen might have an exact measurement of 14.32 feet, and the most useful measurement needed to buy tile could be estimating this quantity to be 14.5 feet. If the kitchen was rectangular and the other side measured 10.9 feet, Bryan might round the other side to 11 feet. Therefore, Bryan would find the total tile necessary according to the following area calculation: $14.5 \times 11 = 159.5$ square feet. To make sure he purchases enough tile, Bryan would probably want to purchase at least 160 square feet of tile. This is a scenario in which an estimation might be more useful than an exact calculation. Having more tile than necessary is better than having an exact amount, in case any tiles are broken or otherwise unusable.

Finally, estimation is helpful when exact answers are necessary. Consider a situation in which Sabina has many operations to perform on numbers with decimals, and she is allowed a calculator to find the result. Even though an exact result can be obtained with a calculator, there is always a possibility that Sabina could make an error while inputting the data. For example, she could miss a decimal place, or misuse a parenthesis, causing a problem with the actual order of operations. In this case, a quick estimation at the beginning would be helpful to make sure the final answer is given with the correct number of units. Sabina has to find the exact total of 10 cars listed for sale at the dealership. Each price has two decimal places included to account for both dollars and cents. If one car is listed at $21, 234.43 but Sabina incorrectly inputs into the calculator the price of $2,123.443, this error would throw off the final sum by almost $20,000. A quick estimation at the beginning, by rounding each price to the nearest thousands place and finding the sum of the prices, would give Sabina an amount to compare the exact amount to. This comparison would let Sabina see if an error was made in her exact calculation.

Solving Real-World Problems Involving Proportions

Fractions appear in everyday situations, and in many scenarios, they appear in the real-world as ratios and in proportions. A **ratio** is formed when two different quantities are compared. For example, in a group of 50 people, if there are 33 females and 17 males, the ratio of females to males is 33 to 17. This expression can be written in the fraction form, $\frac{33}{17}$, or by using the ratio symbol, 33:17. The order of the number matters when forming ratios. In the same setting, the ratio of males to females is 17 to 33, which is equivalent to $\frac{17}{33}$ or 17:33. A **proportion** is an equation involving two ratios. The equation $\frac{a}{b} = \frac{c}{d}$, or $a{:}b = c{:}d$ is a proportion, for real numbers a, b, c, and d. Usually, in one ratio, one of the quantities is unknown, and cross-multiplication is used to solve for the unknown. Consider $\frac{1}{4} = \frac{x}{5}$. To solve for x, cross-multiply to obtain $5 = 4x$. Divide each side by 4 to obtain the solution $x = \frac{5}{4}$. It is also true that percentages are ratios in which the second term is 100. For example, 65% is 65:100 or $\frac{65}{100}$. Therefore, when working with percentages, one is also working with ratios.

Real-world problems frequently involve proportions. For example, consider the following problem: If 2 out of 50 pizzas are usually delivered late from a local Italian restaurant, how many would be late out of 235 orders? The following proportion would be solved with x as the unknown quantity of late pizzas: $\frac{2}{50} = \frac{x}{235}$. Cross multiplying results in $470 = 50x$. Divide both sides by 50 to obtain $x = \frac{470}{50}$, which in lowest terms is equal to $\frac{47}{5}$. In decimal form, this improper fraction is equal to 9.4. Because it does not make sense to answer this question with decimals (portions of pizzas do not get delivered) the answer must be rounded.

Traditional rounding rules would say that 9 pizzas would be expected to be delivered late. However, to be safe, rounding up to 10 pizzas out of 235 would probably make more sense.

Solving Real-World Problems Involving Ratios and Rates of Change

Recall that a **ratio** is the comparison of two different quantities. Comparing 2 apples to 3 oranges results in the ratio 2:3, which can be expressed as the fraction $\frac{2}{3}$. Note that order is important when discussing ratios. The number mentioned first is the numerator, and the number mentioned second is the denominator. The ratio 2:3 does not mean the same quantity as the ratio 3:2. Also, it is important to make sure than when discussing ratios that have units attached to them, the two quantities use the same units. For example, to think of 8 feet to 4 yards, it would make sense to convert 4 yards to feet by multiplying by 3. Therefore, the ratio would be 8 feet to 12 feet, which can be expressed as the fraction $\frac{8}{12}$. Also, note that it is proper to refer to ratios in lowest terms. Therefore, the ratio of 8 feet to 4 yards is equivalent to the fraction $\frac{2}{3}$. Many real-world problems involve ratios. Often, problems with ratios involve proportions, as when two ratios are set equal to find the missing amount. However, some problems involve deciphering single ratios. For example, consider an amusement park that sold 345 tickets last Saturday. If 145 tickets were sold to adults and the rest of the tickets were sold to children, what would the ratio of the number of adult tickets to children's tickets be? A common mistake would be to say the ratio is 145:345. However, 345 is the total number of tickets sold. There were 345 − 145 = 200 tickets sold to children. The correct ratio of adult to children's tickets is 145:200. As a fraction, this expression is written as $\frac{145}{200}$, which can be reduced to $\frac{29}{40}$.

While a ratio compares two measurements using the same units, rates compare two measurements with different units. Examples of rates would be $200 of work for 8 hours, or 500 miles per 20 gallons. Because the units are different, it is important to always include the units when discussing rates. Rates can be easily seen because if they are expressed in words, the two quantities are usually split up using one of the following words: *for, per, on, from, in*. Just as with ratios, it is important to write rates in lowest terms. A common rate that can be found in many real-life situations is cost per unit. This quantity describes how much one item or one unit costs. This rate allows the best buy to be determined, given a couple of different sizes of an item with different costs. For example, if 2 quarts of soup was sold for $3.50 and 3 quarts was sold for $4.60, to determine the best buy, the cost per quart should be found. $\frac{\$3.50}{2} = \$1.75$ per quart, and $\frac{\$4.60}{3} = \$1.53$ per quart. Therefore, the better deal would be the 3-quart option.

Rate of change problems involve calculating a quantity per some unit of measurement. Usually the unit of measurement is time. For example, meters per second is a common rate of change. To calculate this measurement, find the amount traveled in meters and divide by total time traveled. The calculation is an average of the speed over the entire time interval. Another common rate of change used in the real world is miles per hour. Consider the following problem that involves calculating an average rate of change in temperature. Last Saturday, the temperature at 1:00 a.m. was 34 degrees Fahrenheit, and at noon, the temperature had increased to 75 degrees Fahrenheit. What was the average rate of change over that time interval? The average rate of change is calculated by finding the change in temperature and dividing by the total hours elapsed. Therefore, the rate of change was equal to $\frac{75-34}{12-1} = \frac{41}{11}$ degrees per hour. This quantity rounded to two decimal places is equal to 3.72 degrees per hour.

A common rate of change that appears in algebra is the slope calculation. Given a linear equation in one variable, $y = mx + b$, the **slope**, m, is equal to $\frac{rise}{run}$ or $\frac{change\ in\ y}{change\ in\ x}$. In other words, slope is equivalent to the ratio of the vertical and horizontal changes between any two points on a line. The vertical change is known as the **rise,** and the horizontal change is known as the **run.** Given any two points on a line (x_1, y_1) and (x_2, y_2), slope can be calculated with the formula:

$$m = \frac{y_2 - y_1}{x_2 - x_1} = \frac{\Delta y}{\Delta x}$$

Common real-world applications of slope include determining how steep a staircase should be, calculating how steep a road is, and determining how to build a wheelchair ramp.

Many times, problems involving rates and ratios involve proportions. A proportion states that two ratios (or rates) are equal. The property of cross products can be used to determine if a proportion is true, meaning both ratios are equivalent. If $\frac{a}{b} = \frac{c}{d}$, then to clear the fractions, multiply both sides times the least common denominator, bd. This results in $ac = cd$, which is equal to the result of multiplying along both diagonals. For example, $\frac{4}{40} = \frac{1}{10}$ grants the cross product $4 \cdot 10 = 40 \cdot 1$. $40 = 40$ shows that this proportion is true. Cross products are used when proportions are involved in real-world problems. Consider the following: If 3 pounds of fertilizer will cover 75 square feet of grass, how many pounds are needed for 375 square feet? To solve this problem, a proportion can be set up using two ratios. Let x equal the unknown quantity, pounds needed for 375 feet. Then, the equation found by setting the two given ratios equal to one another is $\frac{3}{75} = \frac{x}{375}$. Cross multiplication gives $3 \cdot 375 = 75x$. Therefore, $1{,}125 = 75x$. Divide both sides by 75 to get $x = 15$. Therefore, 15 gallons of fertilizer is needed to cover 75 square feet of grass.

Another application of proportions involves similar triangles. If two triangles have the same measurement as two triangles in another triangle, the triangles are said to be **similar.** If two are the same, the third pair of angles are equal as well because the sum of all angles in a triangle is equal to 180 degrees. Each pair of equivalent angles are known as **corresponding angles. Corresponding sides** face the corresponding angles, and it is true that corresponding sides are in proportion. For example, consider the following set of similar triangles:

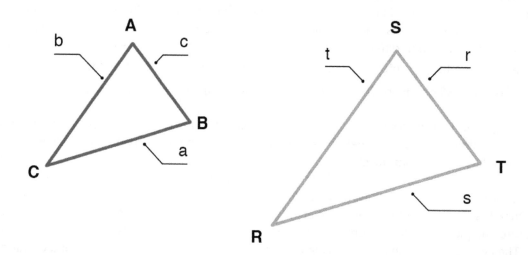

Angles A and R have the same measurement, angles C and T have the same measurement, and angles B and S have the same measurement. Therefore, the following proportion can be set up from the sides:

$$\frac{c}{t} = \frac{a}{r} = \frac{b}{s}$$

This proportion can be helpful in finding missing lengths in pairs of similar triangles. For example, if the following triangles are similar, a proportion can be used to find the missing side lengths, *a* and *b*.

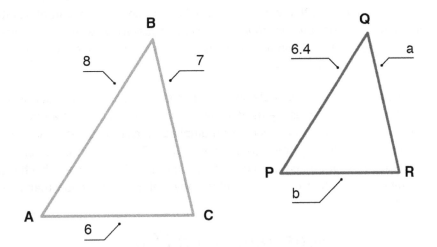

The proportions $\frac{8}{6.4} = \frac{6}{b}$ and $\frac{8}{6.4} = \frac{7}{a}$ can both be cross multiplied and solved to obtain *a* = 5.6 and *b* = 4.8.

A real-life situation that uses similar triangles involves measuring shadows to find heights of unknown objects. Consider the following problem: A building casts a shadow that is 120 feet long, and at the same time, another building that is 80 feet high casts a shadow that is 60 feet long. How tall is the first building? Each building, together with the sun rays and shadows casted on the ground, forms a triangle. They are similar because each building forms a right angle with the ground, and the sun rays form equivalent angles. Therefore, these two pairs of angles are both equal. Because all angles in a triangle add up to 180 degrees, the third angles are equal as well. Both shadows form corresponding sides of the triangle, the buildings form corresponding sides, and the sun rays form corresponding sides. Therefore, the triangles are similar, and the following proportion can be used to find the missing building length:

$$\frac{120}{x} = \frac{60}{80}$$

Cross-multiply to obtain the cross products, 9600 = 60*x*. Then, divide both sides by 60 to obtain *x* = 160. This solution means that the other building is 160 feet high.

Translating Phrases and Sentences into Expressions, Equations, and Inequalities

When presented with a real-world problem that must be solved, the first step is always to determine what the unknown quantity is that must be solved for. Use a variable, such as *x* or *t*, to represent that unknown quantity. Sometimes there can be two or more unknown quantities. In this case, either choose an additional variable, or if a relationship exists between the unknown quantities, express the other quantities in terms of the original variable. After choosing the variables, form algebraic expressions and/or equations that represent the verbal statement in the problem. The following table shows examples of vocabulary used to represent the different operations.

Addition	Sum, plus, total, increase, more than, combined, in all
Subtraction	Difference, less than, subtract, reduce, decrease, fewer, remain
Multiplication	Product, multiply, times, part of, twice, triple
Division	Quotient, divide, split, each, equal parts, per, average, shared

The combination of operations and variables form both mathematical expression and equations. The difference between expressions and equations are that there is no equals sign in an expression, and that expressions are evaluated to find an unknown quantity, while equations are solved to find an unknown quantity. Also, inequalities can exist within verbal mathematical statements. Instead of a statement of equality, expressions state quantities are *less than, less than or equal to, greater than,* or *greater than or equal to.* Another type of inequality is when a quantity is said to be *not equal to* another quantity. The symbol used to represent "not equal to" is $\neq$.

The steps for solving inequalities in one variable are the same steps for solving equations in one variable. The addition and multiplication principles are used. However, to maintain a true statement when using the $<, \leq, >$, and $\geq$ symbols, if a negative number is either multiplied times both sides of an inequality or divided from both sides of an inequality, the sign must be flipped. For instance, consider the following inequality: $3 - 5x \leq 8$. First, 3 is subtracted from each side to obtain $-5x \leq 5$. Then, both sides are divided by -5, while flipping the sign, to obtain $x \geq -1$. Therefore, any real number greater than or equal to -1 satisfies the original inequality.

Measurement and Data

Interpreting Relevant Information from Tables, Charts, and Graphs

Tables, charts, and graphs can be used to convey information about different variables. They are all used to organize, categorize, and compare data, and they all come in different shapes and sizes. Each type has its own way of showing information, whether it is in a column, shape, or picture. To answer a question relating to a table, chart, or graph, some steps should be followed. First, the problem should be read thoroughly to determine what is being asked to determine what quantity is unknown. Then, the title of the table, chart, or graph should be read. The title should clarify what actual data is being summarized in the table. Next, look at the key and both the horizontal and vertical axis labels, if they are given. These items will provide information about how the data is organized. Finally, look to see if there is any more labeling inside the table. Taking the time to get a good idea of what the table is summarizing will be helpful as it is used to interpret information.

Tables are a good way of showing a lot of information in a small space. The information in a table is organized in columns and rows. For example, a table may be used to show the number of votes each candidate received in an election. By interpreting the table, one may observe which candidate won the election and which candidates came in second and third. In using a bar chart to display monthly rainfall amounts in different countries, rainfall can be compared between countries at different times of the year. Graphs are also a useful way to show change in variables over time, as in a line graph, or percentages of a whole, as in a pie graph.

The table below relates the number of items to the total cost. The table shows that 1 item costs $5. By looking at the table further, 5 items cost $25, 10 items cost $50, and 50 items cost $250. This cost can be extended for any number of items. Since 1 item costs $5, then 2 items would cost $10. Though this information isn't in the table, the given price can be used to calculate unknown information.

Number of Items	1	5	10	50
Cost ($)	5	25	50	250

A **bar graph** is a graph that summarizes data using bars of different heights. It is useful when comparing two or more items or when seeing how a quantity changes over time. It has both a horizontal and vertical axis. Interpreting bar graphs includes recognizing what each bar represents and connecting that to the two variables. The bar graph below shows the scores for six people on three different games. The color of the bar shows which game each person played, and the height of the bar indicates their score for that game. William scored 25 on game 3, and Abigail scored 38 on game 3. By comparing the bars, it's obvious that Williams scored lower than Abigail.

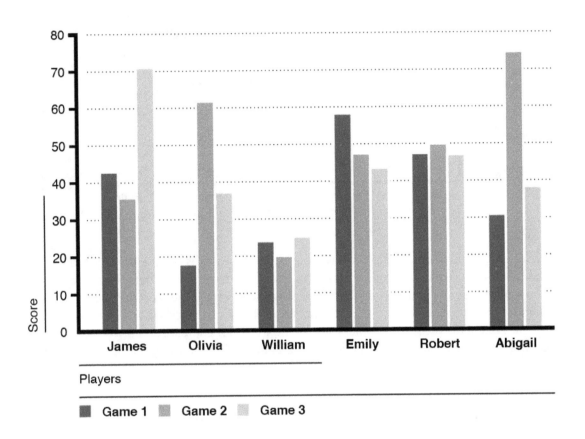

A **line graph** is a way to compare two variables. Each variable is plotted along an axis, and the graph contains both a horizontal and a vertical axis. On a line graph, the line indicates a continuous change. The change can be seen in how the line rises or falls, known as its slope, or rate of change. Often, in line graphs, the horizontal axis represents a variable of time. Audiences can quickly see if an amount has grown or decreased over time. The bottom of the graph, or the x-axis, shows the units for time, such as days, hours, months, etc. If there are multiple lines, a comparison can be made between what the two lines represent. For example, the following line graph shows the change in temperature over five days. The top line represents the high, and the bottom line represents the low for each day. Looking at the top line alone, the high decreases for a day, then increases on Wednesday. Then it decreased on Thursday and increases again on Friday. The low temperatures have a similar trend, shown in bottom line. The range in temperatures each day can also be calculated by finding the difference between the top line and bottom line on a particular day. On Wednesday, the range was 14 degrees, from 62 to 76° F.

Daily Temperatures

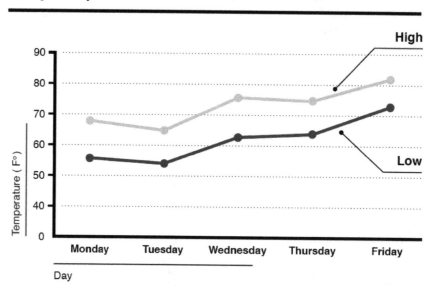

Pie charts are used to show percentages of a whole, as each category is given a piece of the pie, and together all the pieces make up a whole. They are a circular representation of data which are used to highlight numerical proportion. It is true that the arc length of each pie slice is proportional to the amount it individually represents. When a pie chart is shown, an audience can quickly make comparisons by comparing the sizes of the pieces of the pie. They can be useful for comparison between different categories. The following pie chart is a simple example of three different categories shown in comparison to each other.

Light gray represents cats, dark gray represents dogs, and the gray between those two represents other pets. As the pie is cut into three equal pieces, each value represents just more than 33 percent, or $\frac{1}{3}$ of the whole. Values 1 and 2 may be combined to represent $\frac{2}{3}$ of the whole. In an example where the total pie represents 75,000 animals, then cats would be equal to $\frac{1}{3}$ of the total, or 25,000. Dogs would equal 25,000 and other pets would hold equal 25,000.

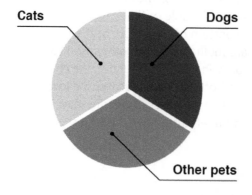

The fact that a circle is 360 degrees is used to create a pie chart. Because each piece of the pie is a percentage of a whole, that percentage is multiplied times 360 to get the number of degrees each piece represents. In the example above, each piece is 1/3 of the whole, so each piece is equivalent to 120 degrees. Together, all three pieces add up to 360 degrees.

Stacked bar graphs, also used fairly frequently, are used when comparing multiple variables at one time. They combine some elements of both pie charts and bar graphs, using the organization of bar graphs and the proportionality aspect of pie charts. The following is an example of a stacked bar graph that represents the number of students in a band playing drums, flutes, trombones, and clarinets. Each bar graph is broken up further into girls and boys.

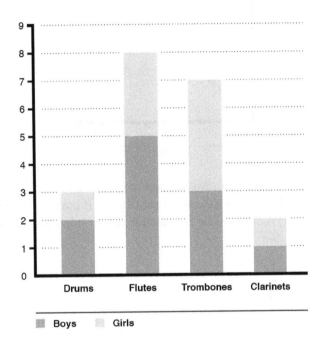

To determine how many boys play tuba, refer to the darker portion of the trombone bar, resulting in 3 students.

A **scatterplot** is another way to represent paired data. It uses Cartesian coordinates, like a line graph, meaning it has both a horizontal and vertical axis. Each data point is represented as a dot on the graph. The dots are never connected with a line. For example, the following is a scatterplot showing people's weight versus height.

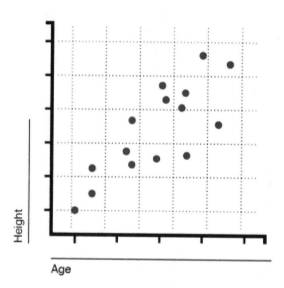

A scatterplot, also known as a **scattergram,** can be used to predict another value and to see if an association, known as a **correlation,** exists between a set of data. If the data resembles a straight line, the data is **associated.** The following is an example of a scatterplot in which the data does not seem to have an association:

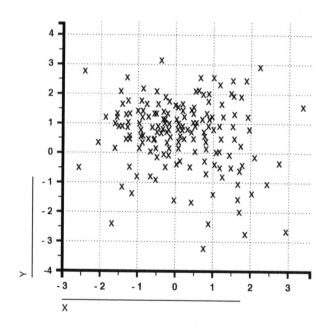

Sets of numbers and other similarly organized data can also be represented graphically. Venn diagrams are a common way to do so. A **Venn diagram** represents each set of data as a circle. The circles overlap, showing that each set of data is overlapping. A Venn diagram is also known as a **logic diagram** because it visualizes all possible logical combinations between two sets. Common elements of two sets are represented by the area of overlap. The following is an example of a Venn diagram of two sets A and B:

Parts of the Venn Diagram

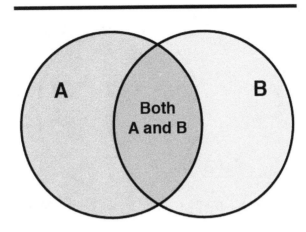

Another name for the area of overlap is the **intersection.** The intersection of A and B, $A \cap B$, contains all elements that are in both sets A and B. The **union** of A and B, $A \cup B$, contains all elements that are in either set A or set B. Finally, the **complement** of $A \cup B$ is equal to all elements that are not in either set A or set B. These elements are placed outside of the circles.

The following is an example of a Venn diagram in which 22 students were surveyed asking about their siblings. Ten students only had a brother, 7 students only had a sister, and 5 had both a brother and a sister. This number 5 is the intersection and is placed where the circles overlap. Two students did not have a brother or a sister. Eight is therefore the complement and is placed outside of the circles.

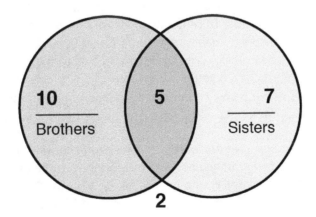

Venn diagrams can have more than two sets of data. The more circles, the more logical combinations are represented by the overlapping. The following is a Venn diagram that represents favorite colors. There were 30 students surveyed. The innermost region represents those students that have a cat, bird, and dog.

Therefore, 2 students had all three. In this example, all students had at least one pet, so no one exists in the complement.

30 students

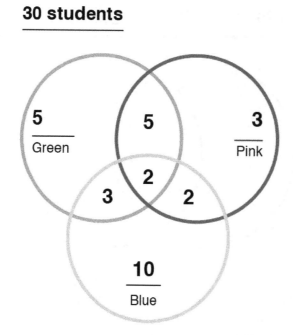

Venn diagrams are typically not drawn to scale, but if they are and their area is proportional to the amount of data it represents, it is known as an **area-proportional Venn diagram**.

Evaluating the Information in Tables, Charts, and Graphs Using Statistics

One way information can be interpreted from tables, charts, and graphs is through statistics. The three most common calculations for a set of data are the mean, median, and mode. These three are called **measures of central tendency**. Measures of central tendency are helpful in comparing two or more different sets of data. The **mean** refers to the average and is found by adding up all values and dividing the total by the number of values. In other words, the mean is equal to the sum of all values divided by the number of data entries. For example, if you bowled a total of 532 points in 4 bowling games, your mean score was $\frac{532}{4} = 133$ points per game. A common application of mean useful to students is calculating what he or she needs to receive on a final exam to receive a desired grade in a class.

The *median* is found by lining up values from least to greatest and choosing the middle value. If there's an even number of values, then the mean of the two middle amounts must be calculated to find the median. For example, the median of the set of dollar amounts $5, $6, $9, $12, and $13 is $9. The **median** of the set of dollar amounts $1, $5, $6, $8, $9, $10 is $7, which is the mean of $6 and $8. The **mode** is the value that occurs the most. The mode of the data set {1, 3, 1, 5, 5, 8, 10} actually refers to two numbers: 1 and 5. In this case, the data set is bimodal because it has two modes. A data set can have no mode if no amount is repeated. Another useful statistic is range. The **range** for a set of data refers to the difference between the highest and lowest value.

In some cases, some numbers in a list of data might have weights attached to them. In that case, a weighted mean can be calculated. A common application of a weighted mean is GPA. In a semester, each class is assigned a number of credit hours, its weight, and at the end of the semester each student receives a grade. To compute GPA, an A is a 4, a B is a 3, a C is a 2, a D is a 1, and an F is a 0. Consider a student that takes a 4-hour English class, a 3-hour math class, and a 4-hour history class and receives all B's. The weighted mean, GPA, is found by multiplying each grade times its weight, number of credit hours, and dividing by the total number of credit hours. Therefore, the student's GPA is:

$$\frac{3 \cdot 4 + 3 \cdot 3 + 3 \cdot 4}{11} = \frac{33}{1} = 3.0.$$

The following bar chart shows how many students attend a cycle on each day of the week. To find the mean attendance for the week, each day's attendance can be added together, $10 + 7 + 6 + 9 + 8 + 14 + 4 = 58$, and the total divided by the number of days, $58 \div 7 = 8.3$. The mean attendance for the week was 8.3 people. The median attendance can be found by putting the attendance numbers in order from least to greatest: 4, 6, 7, 8, 9, 10, 14, and choosing the middle number: 8 people. The mode for attendance is none for this set of data because no numbers repeat. The range is 10, which is found by finding the difference between the lowest number, 4, and the highest number, 14.

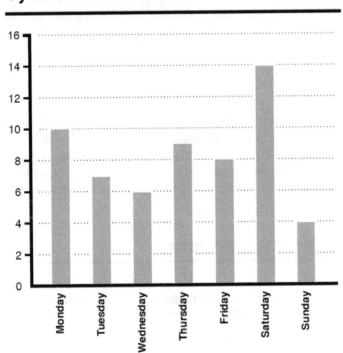

A **histogram** is a bar graph used to group data into "bins" that cover a range on the horizontal, or x-axis. Histograms consist of rectangles whose height is equal to the frequency of a specific category. The horizontal axis represents the specific categories. Because they cover a range of data, these bins have no gaps between bars, unlike the bar graph above. In a histogram showing the heights of adult golden retrievers, the bottom axis would be groups of heights, and the y-axis would be the number of dogs in each range. Evaluating this histogram would show the height of most golden retrievers as falling within a certain range. It also provides information to find the average height and range for how tall golden retrievers may grow.

The following is a histogram that represents exam grades in a given class. The horizontal axis represents ranges of the number of points scored, and the vertical axis represents the number of students. For example, approximately 33 students scored in the 60 to 70 range.

Results of the exam

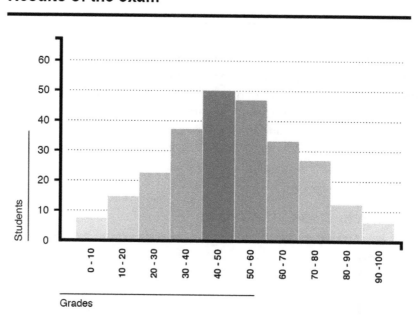

Measures of central tendency can be discussed using a histogram. If the points scored were shown with individual rectangles, the tallest rectangle would represent the mode. A bimodal set of data would have two peaks of equal height. Histograms can be classified as having data **skewed to the left, skewed to the right,** or **normally distributed**, which is also known as **bell-shaped**. These three classifications can be seen in the following chart:

Measures of central tendency images

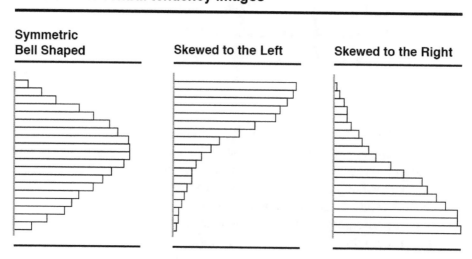

When the data is normal, the mean, median, and mode are all very close. They all represent the most typical value in the data set. The mean is typically used as the best measure of central tendency in this case because it does include all data points. However, if the data is skewed, the mean becomes less meaningful. The median is the best measure of central tendency because it is not affected by any outliers, unlike the mean. When the data is skewed, the mean is dragged in the direction of the skew. Therefore, if the data is not normal, it is best to use the median as the measure of central tendency.

The measures of central tendency and the range may also be found by evaluating information on a line graph.

In the line graph from a previous example that showed the daily high and low temperatures, the average high temperature can be found by gathering data from each day on the triangle line. The days' highs are 82, 78, 75, 65, and 70. The average is found by adding them together to get 370, then dividing by 5 (because there are 5 temperatures). The average high for the five days is 74. If 74 degrees is found on the graph, then it falls in the middle of the values on the triangle line. The mean low temperature can be found in the same way.

Given a set of data, the **correlation coefficient**, r, measures the association between all the data points. If two values are correlated, there is an association between them. However, correlation does not necessarily mean causation, or that that one value causes the other. There is a common mistake made that assumes correlation implies causation. Average daily temperature and number of sunbathers are both correlated and have causation. If the temperature increases, that change in weather causes more people to want to catch some rays. However, wearing plus-size clothing and having heart disease are two variables that are correlated but do not have causation. The larger someone is, the more likely he or she is to have heart disease. However, being overweight does not cause someone to have the disease.

Explaining the Relationship between Two Variables

Independent and dependent are two types of variables that describe how they relate to each other. The **independent variable** is the variable controlled by the experimenter. It stands alone and isn't changed by other parts of the experiment. This variable is normally represented by x and is found on the horizontal, or x-axis, of a graph. The **dependent variable** changes in response to the independent variable. It reacts to, or depends on, the independent variable. This variable is normally represented by y and is found on the vertical, or y-axis of the graph.

The relationship between two variables, x and y, can be seen on a scatterplot.

The following scatterplot shows the relationship between weight and height. The graph shows the weight as x and the height as y. The first dot on the left represents a person who is 45 kg and approximately 150 cm tall. The other dots correspond in the same way. As the dots move to the right and weight increases, height also increases. A line could be drawn through the middle of the dots to move from bottom left to top right. This line would indicate a **positive correlation** between the variables. If the variables had a **negative correlation**, then the dots would move from the top left to the bottom right.

Height and Weight

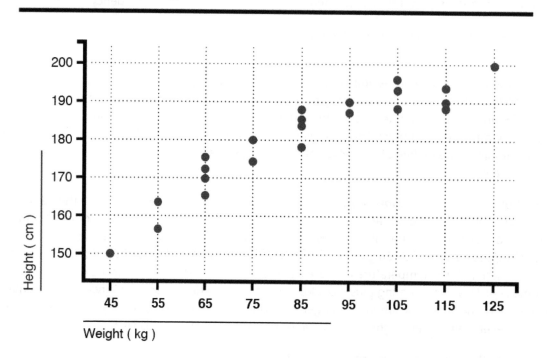

A **scatterplot** is useful in determining the relationship between two variables, but it's not required. Consider an example where a student scores a different grade on his math test for each week of the month. The independent variable would be the weeks of the month. The dependent variable would be the grades, because they change depending on the week. If the grades trended up as the weeks passed, then the relationship between grades and time would be positive. If the grades decreased as the time passed, then the relationship would be negative. (As the number of weeks went up, the grades went down.)

The relationship between two variables can further be described as strong or weak. The relationship between age and height shows a strong positive correlation because children grow taller as they grow up. In adulthood, the relationship between age and height becomes weak, and the dots will spread out. People stop growing in adulthood, and their final heights vary depending on factors like genetics and health. The closer the dots on the graph, the stronger the relationship. As they spread apart, the relationship becomes weaker. If they are too spread out to determine a correlation up or down, then the variables are said to have no correlation.

Variables are values that change, so determining the relationship between them requires an evaluation of who changes them. If the variable changes because of a result in the experiment, then it's dependent. If the variable changes before the experiment, or is changed by the person controlling the experiment, then it's the independent variable. As they interact, one is manipulated by the other. The manipulator is the independent, and the manipulated is the dependent. Once the independent and dependent variable are determined, they can be evaluated to have a positive, negative, or no correlation.

Calculating Geometric Quantities

Perimeter and area are two commonly used geometric quantities that describe objects. **Perimeter** is the distance around an object. The perimeter of an object can be found by adding the lengths of all sides. Perimeter may be used in problems dealing with lengths around objects such as fences or borders. It may also be used in finding missing lengths, or working backwards. If the perimeter is given, but a length is missing, use subtraction to find the missing length. Given a square with side length s, the formula for perimeter is $P = 4s$. Given a rectangle with length l and width w, the formula for perimeter is $P = 2l + 2w$. The perimeter of a triangle is found by adding the three side lengths, and the perimeter of a trapezoid is found by adding the four side lengths. The units for perimeter are always the original units of length, such as meters, inches, miles, etc. When discussing a circle, the distance around the object is referred to as its circumference, not perimeter. The formula for circumference of a circle is $C = 2\pi r$, where r represents the radius of the circle. This formula can also be written as $C = d\mu$, where d represents the diameter of the circle.

Area is the two-dimensional space covered by an object. These problems may include the area of a rectangle, a yard, or a wall to be painted. Finding the area may be a simple formula, or it may require multiple formulas to be used together. The units for area are square units, such as square meters, square inches, and square miles. Given a square with side length s, the formula for its area is $A = s^2$. Some other formulas for common shapes are shown below.

Shape	Formula	Graphic
Rectangle	$Area = length \times width$	
Triangle	$Area = \dfrac{1}{2} \times base \times height$	
Circle	$Area = \pi \times radius^2$	

The following formula, not as widely used as those shown above, but very important, is the area of a trapezoid:

Area of a Trapezoid

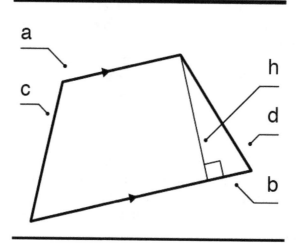

$$A = \frac{1}{2}\,(\,a + b\,)\,h$$

While some geometric figures may be given as pictures, others may be described in words. If a rectangular playing field with dimensions 95 meters long by 50 meters wide is measured for perimeter, the distance around the field must be found. The perimeter includes two lengths and two widths to measure the entire outside of the field. This quantity can be calculated using the following equation:

$$P = 2(95) + 2(50) = 290\ m$$

The distance around the field is 290 meters.

Perimeter and area are two-dimensional descriptions; volume is three-dimensional. **Volume** describes the amount of space that an object occupies, but it's different from area because it has three dimensions instead of two. The units for volume are cubic units, such as cubic meters, cubic inches, and cubic miles. Volume can be found by using formulas for common objects such as cylinders and boxes.

To find the area of the shapes above, use the given dimensions of the shape in the formula. Complex shapes might require more than one formula. To find the area of the figure below, break the figure into two shapes. The rectangle has dimensions 11 cm by 6 cm. The triangle has dimensions 3 cm by 6 cm. Plug the dimensions into the rectangle formula: $A = 11 \times 6$. Multiplication yields an area of 66 cm². The triangle area can be found using the formula:

$$A = \frac{1}{2} \times 4 \times 6$$

Multiplication yields an area of 12 cm². Add the areas of the two shapes to find the total area of the figure, which is 78 cm².

Instead of combining areas, some problems may require subtracting them, or finding the difference.

To find the area of the shaded region in the figure below, determine the area of the whole figure. Then the area of the circle can be subtracted from the whole.

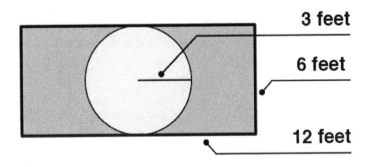

The following formula shows the area of the outside rectangle:

$$A = 12 \times 6 = 72 \; ft^2$$

The area of the inside circle can be found by the following formula:

$$A = \pi r^2 = \pi(3^2)$$

$$9\pi = 28.27 \, ft^2$$

As the shaded area is outside the circle, the area for the circle can be subtracted from the area of the rectangle to yield an area of $43.73 \, ft^2$.

The following chart shows a diagram and formula for the volume of two objects.

Shape	Formula	Diagram
Rectangular Prism (box)	$V = length \times width \times height$	
Cylinder	$V = \pi \times radius^2 \times height$	

Volume formulas of these two objects are derived by finding the area of the bottom two-dimensional shape, such as the circle or rectangle, and then multiplying times the height of the three-dimensional shape. Other volume formulas include the volume of a cube with side length s: $V = s^3$; the volume of a sphere with radius r: $V = \frac{4}{3}\pi r^3$; and the volume of a cone with radius r and height h.

$$V = \frac{1}{3}\pi r^2 h$$

If a soda can has a height of 5 inches and a radius on the top of 1.5 inches, the volume can be found using one of the given formulas. A soda can is a cylinder. Knowing the given dimensions, the formula can be completed as follows:

$$V = \pi \, (radius)^2 \times height$$

$$\pi \, (1.5)^2 \times 5 = 35.325 \, inches^3$$

Notice that the units for volume are inches cubed because it refers to the number of cubic inches required to fill the can.

With any geometric calculations, it's important to determine what dimensions are given and what quantities the problem is asking for. If a connection can be made between them, the answer can be found.

Other geometric quantities can include angles inside a triangle. The sum of the measures of three angles in any triangle is 180 degrees. Therefore, if only two angles are known inside a triangle, the third can be found by subtracting the sum of the two known quantities from 180. Two angles whose sum is equal to 90 degrees are known as **complementary angles**. For example, angles measuring 72 and 18 degrees are complementary, and each angle is a complement of the other. Finally, two angles whose sum is equal to 180 degrees are known as **supplementary angles.** To find the supplement of an angle, subtract the given angle from 180 degrees. For example, the supplement of an angle that is 50 degrees is 180 − 50 = 130 degrees.

These terms involving angles can be seen in many types of word problems. For example, consider the following problem: The measure of an angle is 60 degrees less than two times the measure of its complement. What is the angle's measure? To solve this, let x be the unknown angle. Therefore, its complement is 90 − x. The problem gives that:

$$x = 2(90 - x) - 60$$

To solve for x, distribute the 2, and collect like terms. This process results in $x = 120 - 2x$. Then, use the addition property to add $2x$ to both sides to obtain $3x = 120$. Finally, use the multiplication properties of equality to divide both sides by 3 to get $x = 40$. Therefore, the angle measures 40 degrees. Also, its complement measures 50 degrees.

Converting Within and Between Standard and Metric Systems

When working with dimensions, sometimes the given units don't match the formula, and conversions must be made. The metric system has base units of meter for length, kilogram for mass, and liter for liquid volume. This system expands to three places above the base unit and three places below. These places correspond with prefixes with a base of 10.

The following table shows the conversions:

kilo-	hecto-	deka-	base	deci-	centi-	milli-
1,000 times the base	100 times the base	10 times the base		1/10 times the base	1/100 times the base	1/1000 times the base

To convert between units within the metric system, values with a base ten can be multiplied. The decimal can also be moved in the direction of the new unit by the same number of zeros on the number. For example, 3 meters is equivalent to .003 kilometers. The decimal moved three places (the same number of zeros for kilo-) to the left (the same direction from base to kilo-). Three meters is also equivalent to 3,000 millimeters. The decimal is moved three places to the right because the prefix milli- is three places to the right of the base unit.

The English Standard system used in the United States has a base unit of foot for length, pound for weight, and gallon for liquid volume. These conversions aren't as easy as the metric system because they aren't a base ten model. The following table shows the conversions within this system.

Length	Weight	Capacity
1 foot (ft) = 12 inches (in) 1 yard (yd) = 3 feet 1 mile (mi) = 5280 feet 1 mile = 1760 yards	1 pound (lb) = 16 ounces (oz) 1 ton = 2000 pounds	1 tablespoon (tbsp) = 3 teaspoons (tsp) 1 cup (c) = 16 tablespoons 1 cup = 8 fluid ounces (oz) 1 pint (pt) = 2 cups 1 quart (qt) = 2 pints 1 gallon (gal) = 4 quarts

When converting within the English Standard system, most calculations include a conversion to the base unit and then another to the desired unit. For example, take the following problem: 3 $quarts$ = ___ $cups$. There is no straight conversion from quarts to cups, so the first conversion is from quarts to pints. There are 2 pints in 1 quart, so there are 6 pints in 3 quarts. This conversion can be solved as a proportion:

$$\frac{3\ qt}{x} = \frac{1\ qt}{2\ pints}$$

It can also be observed as a ratio 2:1, expanded to 6:3. Then the 6 pints must be converted to cups. The ratio of pints to cups is 1:2, so the expanded ratio is 6:12. For 6 pints, the measurement is 12 cups. This problem can also be set up as one set of fractions to cancel out units. It begins with the given information and cancels out matching units on top and bottom to yield the answer. Consider the following expression:

$$\frac{3\ quarts}{1} \times \frac{2\ pints}{1\ quart} \times \frac{2\ cups}{1\ pint}$$

It's set up so that units on the top and bottom cancel each other out:

$$\frac{3\ \cancel{quarts}}{1} \times \frac{2\ \cancel{pints}}{1\ \cancel{quart}} \times \frac{2\ cups}{1\ \cancel{pint}}$$

The numbers can be calculated as 3 × 3 × 2 on the top and 1 on the bottom. It still yields an answer of 12 cups.

This process of setting up fractions and canceling out matching units can be used to convert between standard and metric systems. A few common equivalent conversions are 2.54 cm = 1 inch, 3.28 feet = 1 meter, and 2.205 pounds = 1 kilogram. Writing these as fractions allows them to be used in conversions. For the fill-in-the-blank problem 5 meters = ___ feet, an expression using conversions starts with the expression $\frac{5\ meters}{1} \times \frac{3.28\ feet}{1\ meter}$, where the units of meters will cancel each other out, and the final unit is feet. Calculating the numbers yields 16.4 feet. This problem only required two fractions. Others may require longer expressions, but the underlying rule stays the same. When there's a unit on the top of the fraction that's the same as the unit on the bottom, then they cancel each other out. Using this logic and the conversions given above, many units can be converted between and within the different systems.

The conversion between Fahrenheit and Celsius is found in a formula:

$$°C = (°F - 32) \times \frac{5}{9}$$

For example, to convert 78 °F to Celsius, the given temperature would be entered into the formula:

$$°C = (78 - 32) \times \frac{5}{9}$$

Solving the equation, the temperature comes out to be 25.56°C. To convert in the other direction, the formula becomes:

$$°F = °C * \frac{9}{5} + 32$$

Remember the order of operations when calculating these conversions.

Practice Questions

1. What is $\frac{12}{60}$ converted to a percentage?
    a. 0.20
    b. 20%
    c. 25%
    d. 12%

2. Which of the following is the correct decimal form of the fraction $\frac{14}{33}$ rounded to the nearest hundredth place?
    a. 0.420
    b. 0.42
    c. 0.424
    d. 0.140

3. Which of the following represents the correct sum of $\frac{14}{15}$ and $\frac{2}{5}$?
    a. $\frac{20}{15}$
    b. $\frac{4}{3}$
    c. $\frac{16}{20}$
    d. $\frac{4}{5}$

4. What is the product of $\frac{5}{14}$ and $\frac{7}{20}$?
    a. $\frac{1}{8}$
    b. $\frac{35}{280}$
    c. $\frac{12}{34}$
    d. $\frac{1}{2}$

5. What is the result of dividing 24 by $\frac{8}{5}$?
    a. $\frac{5}{3}$
    b. $\frac{3}{5}$
    c. $\frac{120}{8}$
    d. 15

6. Subtract $\frac{5}{14}$ from $\frac{5}{24}$. Which of the following is the correct result?

  a. $\frac{25}{168}$

  b. 0

  c. $-\frac{25}{168}$

  d. $\frac{1}{10}$

7. Which of the following is a correct mathematical statement?

  a. $\frac{1}{3} < -\frac{4}{3}$

  b. $-\frac{1}{3} > \frac{4}{3}$

  c. $\frac{1}{3} > -\frac{4}{3}$

  d. $-\frac{1}{3} \geq \frac{4}{3}$

8. Which of the following is incorrect?

  a. $-\frac{1}{5} < \frac{4}{5}$

  b. $\frac{4}{5} > -\frac{1}{5}$

  c. $-\frac{1}{5} > \frac{4}{5}$

  d. $\frac{1}{5} > -\frac{4}{5}$

9. What is the solution to the equation $3(x + 2) = 14x - 5$?

  a. $x = 1$

  b. No solution

  c. $x = 0$

  d. All real numbers

10. What is the solution to the equation $10 - 5x + 2 = 7x + 12 - 12x$?

  a. $x = 12$

  b. No solution

  c. $x = 0$

  d. All real numbers

11. Which of the following is the result when solving the equation $4(x + 5) + 6 = 2(2x + 3)$?

  a. Any real number is a solution.

  b. There is no solution.

  c. $x = 6$ is the solution.

  d. $x = 26$ is the solution.

12. How many cases of cola can Lexi purchase if each case is $3.50 and she has $40?
    a. 10
    b. 12
    c. 11.4
    d. 11

13. Two consecutive integers exist such that the sum of three times the first and two less than the second is equal to 411. What are those integers?
    a. 103 and 104
    b. 104 and 105
    c. 102 and 103
    d. 100 and 101

14. In a neighborhood, 15 out of 80 of the households have children under the age of 18. What percentage of the households have children?
    a. 0.1875%
    b. 18.75%
    c. 1.875%
    d. 15%

15. Gina took an algebra test last Friday. There were 35 questions, and she answered 60% of them correctly. How many correct answers did she have?
    a. 35
    b. 20
    c. 21
    d. 25

16. Paul took a written driving test, and he got 12 of the questions correct. If he answered 75% of the total questions correctly, how many problems were there in the test?
    a. 25
    b. 16
    c. 20
    d. 18

17. If a car is purchased for $15,395 with a 7.25% sales tax, how much is the total price?
    a. $15,395.07
    b. $16,511.14
    c. $16,411.13
    d. $15,402

18. A car manufacturer usually makes 15,412 SUVs, 25,815 station wagons, 50,412 sedans, 8,123 trucks, and 18,312 hybrids a month. About how many cars are manufactured each month?
    a. 120,000
    b. 200,000
    c. 300,000
    d. 12,000

19. Each year, a family goes to the grocery store every week and spends $105. About how much does the family spend annually on groceries?

   a. $10,000
   b. $50,000
   c. $500
   d. $5,000

20. Bindee is having a barbeque on Sunday and needs 12 packets of ketchup for every 5 guests. If 60 guests are coming, how many packets of ketchup should she buy?

   a. 100
   b. 12
   c. 144
   d. 60

21. A grocery store sold 48 bags of apples in one day, and 9 of the bags contained Granny Smith apples. The rest contained Red Delicious apples. What is the ratio of bags of Granny Smith to bags of Red Delicious that were sold?

   a. 48:9
   b. 39:9
   c. 9:48
   d. 9:39

22. If Oscar's bank account totaled $4,000 in March and $4,900 in June, what was the rate of change in his bank account total over those three months?

   a. $900 a month
   b. $300 a month
   c. $4,900 a month
   d. $100 a month

23. Erin and Katie work at the same ice cream shop. Together, they always work less than 21 hours a week. In a week, if Katie worked two times as many hours as Erin, how many hours could Erin work?

   a. Less than 7 hours
   b. Less than or equal to 7 hours
   c. More than 7 hours
   d. Less than 8 hours

24. From the chart below, which two are preferred by more men than women?

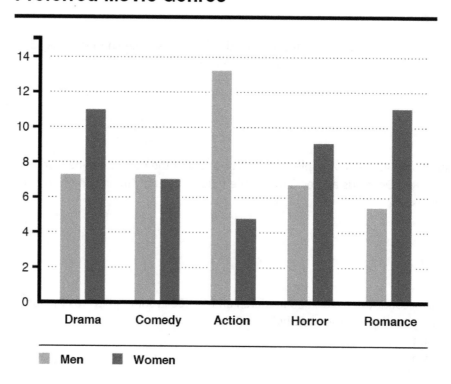

Preferred Movie Genres

 a. Comedy and Action
 b. Drama and Comedy
 c. Action and Horror
 d. Action and Romance

25. Which type of graph best represents a continuous change over a period of time?
 a. Bar graph
 b. Line graph
 c. Pie graph
 d. Histogram

26. Using the graph below, what is the mean number of visitors for the first 4 hours?

Museum Visitors

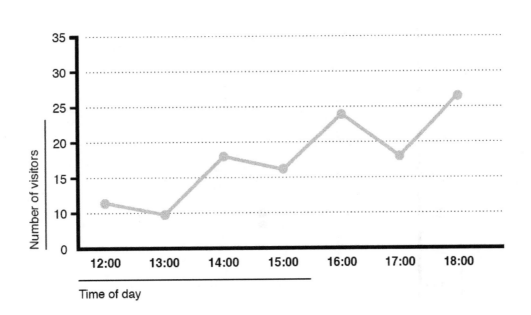

Time of day

a. 12
b. 13
c. 14
d. 15

27. What is the mode for the grades shown in the chart below?

Science Grades	
Jerry	65
Bill	95
Anna	80
Beth	95
Sara	85
Ben	72
Jordan	98

a. 65
b. 33
c. 95
d. 90

28. What type of relationship is there between age and attention span as represented in the graph below?

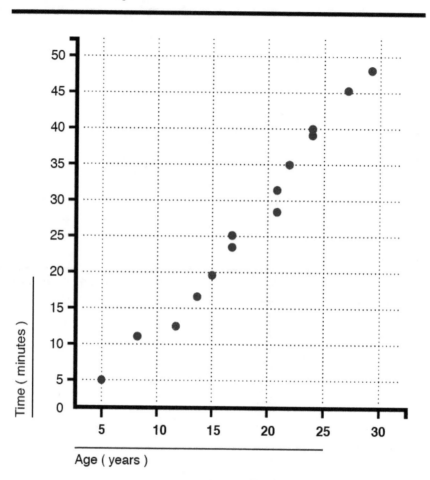

Attention Span

a. No correlation
b. Positive correlation
c. Negative correlation
d. Weak correlation

29. What is the area of the shaded region?

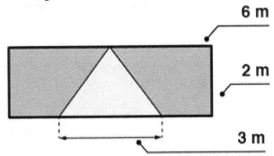

6 m

2 m

3 m

    a. 9 m²
    b. 12 m²
    c. 6 m²
    d. 8 m²

30. What is the volume of the cylinder below?

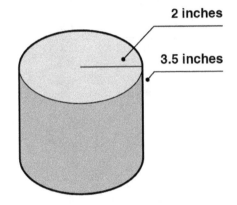

2 inches

3.5 inches

    a. 18.84 in³
    b. 45.00 in³
    c. 70.43 in³
    d. 43.96 in³

31. How many kiloliters are in 6 liters?
    a. 6,000
    b. 600
    c. 0.006
    d. 0.0006

32. How many centimeters are in 3 feet? (Note: 2.54cm = 1 inch)
    a. 0.635
    b. 91.44
    c. 14.17
    d. 7.62

Answer Explanations

1. B: The fraction $\frac{12}{60}$ can be reduced to $\frac{1}{5}$, in lowest terms. First, it must be converted to a decimal. Dividing 1 by 5 results in 0.2. Then, to convert to a percentage, move the decimal point two units to the right and add the percentage symbol. The result is 20%.

2. B: If a calculator is used, divide 33 into 14 and keep two decimal places. If a calculator is not used, multiply both the numerator and denominator times 3. This results in the fraction $\frac{42}{99}$, and hence a decimal of 0.42.

3. B: Common denominators must be used. The LCD is 15, and $\frac{2}{5} = \frac{6}{15}$. Therefore, $\frac{14}{15} + \frac{6}{15} = \frac{20}{15}$, and in lowest terms the answer is $\frac{4}{3}$. A common factor of 5 was divided out of both the numerator and denominator.

4. A: A product is found by multiplication. Multiplying two fractions together is easier when common factors are cancelled first to avoid working with larger numbers

$$\frac{5}{14} \times \frac{7}{20} = \frac{5}{2 \times 7} \times \frac{7}{5 \times 4}$$

$$\frac{1}{2} \times \frac{1}{4} = \frac{1}{8}$$

5. D: Division is completed by multiplying times the reciprocal. Therefore:

$$24 \div \frac{8}{5} = \frac{24}{1} \times \frac{5}{8}$$

$$\frac{3 \times 8}{1} \times \frac{5}{8} = \frac{15}{1} = 15$$

6. C: Common denominators must be used. The LCD is 168, so each fraction must be converted to have 168 as the denominator.

$$\frac{5}{24} - \frac{5}{14} = \frac{5}{24} \times \frac{7}{7} - \frac{5}{14} \times \frac{12}{12}$$

$$\frac{35}{168} - \frac{60}{168} = -\frac{25}{168}$$

7. C: The correct mathematical statement is the one in which the number to the left on the number line is less than the number to the right on the number line. It is written in answer C that $\frac{1}{3} > -\frac{4}{3}$, which is the same as $-\frac{4}{3} < \frac{1}{3}$, a correct statement.

8. C: $-\frac{1}{5} > \frac{4}{5}$ is incorrect. The expression on the left is negative, which means that it is smaller than the expression on the right. As it is written, the inequality states that the expression on the left is greater than the expression on the right, which is not true.

9. A: First, the distributive property must be used on the left side. This results in:

$$3x + 6 = 14x - 5$$

104

The addition property is then used to add 5 to both sides, and then to subtract $3x$ from both sides, resulting in $11 = 11x$. Finally, the multiplication property is used to divide each side by 11. Therefore, $x = 1$ is the solution.

10. D: First, like terms are collected to obtain:

$$12 - 5x = -5x + 12$$

Then, if the addition principle is used to move the terms with the variable, $5x$ is added to both sides and the mathematical statement $12 = 12$ is obtained. This is always true; therefore, all real numbers satisfy the original equation.

11. B: The distributive property is used on both sides to obtain:

$$4x + 20 + 6 = 4x + 6$$

Then, like terms are collected on the left, resulting in:

$$4x + 26 = 4x + 6$$

Next, the addition principle is used to subtract $4x$ from both sides, and this results in the false statement $26 = 6$. Therefore, there is no solution.

12. D: This is a one-step real-world application problem. The unknown quantity is the number of cases of cola to be purchased. Let x be equal to this amount. Because each case costs $3.50, the total number of cases times $3.50 must equal $40. This translates to the mathematical equation $3.5x = 40$. Divide both sides by 3.5 to obtain $x = 11.4286$, which has been rounded to four decimal places. Because cases are sold whole (the store does not sell portions of cases), and there is not enough money to purchase 12 cases, there is only enough money to purchase 11.

13. A: First, the variables have to be defined. Let x be the first integer; therefore, $x + 1$ is the second integer. This is a two-step problem. The sum of three times the first and two less than the second is translated into the following expression:

$$3x + (x + 1 - 2)$$

This expression is set equal to 411 to obtain:

$$3x + (x + 1 - 2) = 412$$

The left-hand side is simplified to obtain $4x - 1 = 411$. The addition and multiplication properties are used to solve for x. First, add 1 to both sides and then divide both sides by 4 to obtain $x = 103$. The next consecutive integer is 104.

14. B: First, the information is translated into the ratio $\frac{15}{80}$. To find the percentage, translate this fraction into a decimal by dividing 15 by 80. The corresponding decimal is 0.1875. Move the decimal point two units to the right to obtain the percentage 18.75%.

15. C: Gina answered 60% of 35 questions correctly; 60% can be expressed as the decimal 0.60. Therefore, she answered $0.60 \times 35 = 21$ questions correctly.

16. B: The unknown quantity is the number of total questions on the test. Let x be equal to this unknown quantity. Therefore, $0.75x = 12$. Divide both sides by 0.75 to obtain $x = 16$.

17. B: If sales tax is 7.25%, the price of the car must be multiplied times 1.0725 to account for the additional sales tax. Therefore:

$$15,395 \times 1.0725 = 16,511.1375$$

This amount is rounded to the nearest cent, which is $16,511.14.

18. A: Rounding can be used to find the best approximation. All of the values can be rounded to the nearest thousand. 15,412 SUVs can be rounded to 15,000. 25,815 station wagons can be rounded to 26,000. 50,412 sedans can be rounded to 50,000. 8,123 trucks can be rounded to 8,000. Finally, 18,312 hybrids can be rounded to 18,000. The sum of the rounded values is 117,000, which is closest to 120,000.

19. D: There are 52 weeks in a year, and if the family spends $105 each week, that amount is close to $100. A good approximation is $100 a week for 50 weeks, which is found through the product $50 \times 100 = \$5,000$.

20. C: This problem involves ratios and percentages. If 12 packets are needed for every 5 people, this statement is equivalent to the ratio $\frac{12}{5}$. The unknown amount x is the number of ketchup packets needed for 60 people. The proportion $\frac{12}{5} = \frac{x}{60}$ must be solved. Cross-multiply to obtain $12 \times 60 = 5x$. Therefore, $720 = 5x$. Divide each side by 5 to obtain $x = 144$.

21. D: There were 48 total bags of apples sold. If 9 bags were Granny Smith and the rest were Red Delicious, then $48 - 9 = 39$ bags were Red Delicious. Therefore, the ratio of Granny Smith to Red Delicious is 9:39.

22. B: The average rate of change is found by calculating the difference in dollars over the elapsed time. Therefore, the rate of change is equal to $4,900-$4,000÷3 months, which is equal to $900÷3 or $300 a month.

23. A: Let x be the unknown, the number of hours Erin can work. We know Katie works $2x$, and the sum of all hours is less than 21. Therefore, $x + 2x < 21$, which simplifies into $3x < 21$. Solving this results in the inequality $x < 7$ after dividing both sides by 3. Therefore, Erin can work less than 7 hours.

24. A: The chart is a bar chart showing how many men and women prefer each genre of movies. The dark gray bars represent the number of women, while the light gray bars represent the number of men. The light gray bars are higher and represent more men than women for the genres of Comedy and Action.

25. B: A line graph represents continuous change over time. The line on the graph is continuous and not broken, as on a scatter plot. A bar graph may show change but isn't necessarily continuous over time. A pie graph is better for representing percentages of a whole. Histograms are best used in grouping sets of data in bins to show the frequency of a certain variable.

26. C: The mean for the number of visitors during the first 4 hours is 14. The mean is found by calculating the average for the four hours. Adding up the total number of visitors during those hours gives $12 + 10 + 18 + 16 = 56$. Then $56 \div 4 = 14$.

27. C: The mode for a set of data is the value that occurs the most. The grade that appears the most is 95. It's the only value that repeats in the set.

28. B: The relationship between age and time for attention span is a positive correlation because the general trend for the data is up and to the right. As the age increases, so does attention span.

29. A: The area of the shaded region is calculated in a few steps. First, the area of the rectangle is found using the formula:

$$A = length \times width = 6 \times 2 = 12$$

Second, the area of the triangle is found using the formula:

$$A = \frac{1}{2} \times base \times height = \frac{1}{2} \times 3 \times 2 = 3$$

The last step is to take the rectangle area and subtract the triangle area. The area of the shaded region is:

$$A = 12 - 3 = 9m^2$$

30. D: The volume for a cylinder is found by using the formula:

$$V = \pi r^2 h = \pi(2^2) \times 3.5 = 43.96 in^3$$

31. C: There are 0.006 kiloliters in 6 liters because 1 liter = 0.001 kiloliters. The conversion comes from the chart where the prefix kilo is found three places to the left of the base unit.

32. B: The conversion between feet and centimeters requires a middle term. As there are 2.54 centimeters in 1 inch, the conversion between inches and feet must be found. As there are 12 inches in a foot, the fractions can be set up as follows:

$$3\ feet \times \frac{12\ inches}{1\ foot} \times \frac{2.54\ cm}{1\ inch}$$

The feet and inches cancel out to leave only centimeters for the answer. The numbers are calculated across the top and bottom to yield:

$$\frac{3 \times 12 \times 2.54}{1 \times 1} = 91.44$$

The number and units used together form the answer of 91.44 cm.

Science

Human Anatomy and Physiology

Humans

Humans are complex organisms. They have many structures and functions that work in conjunction to maintain life. Breaking up the human body into smaller parts makes it easier to understand. **Anatomy** is the study of external and internal body parts and structures, and their physical relationships to each other. **Gross anatomy** is the study of large structures that are visible to the naked eye. **Microscopic anatomy** is the study of structures that can only be seen with the help of magnification, such as under a microscope. **Systemic anatomy** is the study of the major organ systems. **Developmental anatomy** is the study of the physical changes that happen between conception and physical maturity. **Physiology** is the study of the function of living organisms and their body parts. **Pathophysiology** is the study of how diseases affect organs and organ system functions. The human body is made up of different types of cells that join together to form tissues, which then form together to create organs. Organs provide functions for the body that are vital for sustaining life.

Levels of Organization of the Human Body
There are six levels of organization that can help describe the human body. These levels, in smallest to largest size order, are chemical, cellular, tissue, organ, organ system, and organism. The **chemical level** includes atoms and molecules, which are the smallest building blocks of matter. When atoms bind together, they form molecules, which in turn make up chemicals. All body structures are made up of these small elements. **Cells** are the smallest units of living organisms. They function independently to carry out vital functions of every organism. Cells that are similar then bind together to form tissues. **Tissues** perform specific functions by having all of the cells work together. For example, muscle tissue is made up of contractile cells that help the body move. **Organs** are made up of two or more types of tissue and perform physiological functions. **Organ systems** are made up of several organs together that work to perform a major bodily function. **Organisms** include the human body as a whole and all of its structures that perform life-sustaining functions.

There are eleven major organ systems of the human body. The **integumentary system** comprises the skin, hair, and nails, which are all on the outside of the body. It is responsible for enclosing and protecting the internal body structures. It contains many sensory receptors on its surface. The **skeletal system** comprises cartilage, bones, and joints. It supports the body and allows for movement of the body in conjunction with the **muscular system**, which is composed of skeletal muscles and tendons and also helps maintain body temperature. The **nervous system** is made up of the brain, spinal cord, and peripheral nerves. It is in charge of detecting and processing sensory information from the entire body and then sending out an appropriate response, such as taking a hand away quickly after touching something hot.

The **endocrine system** includes the pituitary gland, thyroid gland, pancreas, adrenal glands, the testes in males, and the ovaries in females. It is responsible for regulating most bodily processes and secreting hormones. The **cardiovascular system** comprises the heart and blood vessels. Together, these structures are responsible for taking nutrients and oxygen to all of the tissues in the body. This system also helps regulate body temperature. The **lymphatic system** includes the thymus, lymph nodes, spleen, and lymphatic vessels. It is in charge of returning bodily fluids to the blood and fighting off pathogens that enter the body. The **respiratory system** includes the nasal passage, trachea, and lungs. It works to take in oxygen from the environment and deliver it to the blood and to remove carbon dioxide from the body. The **digestive system** consists of the stomach, liver, gallbladder, large intestine, and small intestine. It processes food and liquid into energy for the body and removes waste from undigested food. The **urinary system** includes the kidneys and urinary bladder. It removes and excretes waste from the blood and controls water balance within the body. The **reproductive system** in males includes the epididymis and testes and in females the mammary glands, ovaries, and uterus. Both the male and female systems produce hormones and gametes. The male system delivers its gametes to females. The female system supports an embryo until birth and then produces milk for the baby.

Body Cavities

Body cavities in humans are the fluid-filled spaces that contain the organs. They are located just under the skin. They provide room for the organs to adjust as the body changes position, and they contain protective membranes. Some cavities contain bones that protect the organs as well. The **dorsal cavity** is located along the posterior, or back, side of the body. It contains the brain and spinal cord in the **cranial cavity** and the **spinal cavity**, respectively, although these two subdivided cavities are continuous. The dorsal cavity contains the **meninges,** which is a multilayered membrane that runs around the brain and spinal cord and helps protect these delicate organs. The cranial cavity is the anterior portion of the dorsal cavity. In addition to the brain, it specifically contains the meninges of the brain and cerebrospinal fluid.

The spinal cavity is the posterior portion of the dorsal cavity and contains the meninges of the spinal cord and the fluid-filled spaces in between the vertebrae, in addition to the spinal cord. This portion of the dorsal cavity is the narrowest of all of the body's cavities. The **ventral cavity** is the interior space in the front of the body, anterior to the dorsal cavity. It comprises the **thoracic** and **abdominopelvic cavities**. The thoracic cavity is located within the rib cage in the chest. It encases the cardiovascular and respiratory system organs, as well as the thymus and esophagus.

Ventral Front

It is lined by two types of membranes: the **pleura,** which is a membrane that goes around the lungs, and the **pericardium**, which is the membrane that lines the outside of the heart. The abdominopelvic cavity is located below the thoracic cavity and underneath the diaphragm. The diaphragm is a sheet of skeletal muscle that is located just beneath the lungs. This cavity contains the organs of the digestive, renal, urinary, and reproductive systems, as well as some endocrine glands. It is lined by a membrane called the **peritoneum**. It can be divided into four quadrants: right upper, right lower, left upper, and left lower.

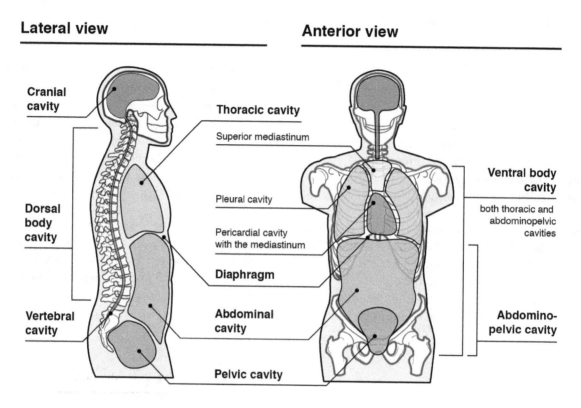

Human Tissues

There are four primary types of **tissue** found in the human body: epithelial, connective, muscle, and neural. Each tissue type has specific characteristics that enable organs and organ systems to function properly. **Epithelial tissue** includes epithelia and glands. **Epithelia** are the layers of cells that cover exposed surfaces and line internal cavities and passageways. The cells are laid out in sheets and have tight cell bonds between them. The three main cell shapes in epithelia are squamous, which appear flattened; cuboidal, which appear as cubes; and columnar, which appear as tall columns. The cell layers can be described as simple, which is when the cells are in one row; stratified, which is when there are multiple rows of cells with only one of the layers connected to the basement membrane and the other layers strongly connected to each other; or pseudostratified, which is when cells are in one row but the nuclei of the cells appear stratified and are not in line with each other.

Epithelia do not contain blood vessels and can often regenerate quickly to replace dead and damaged cells. Since they are avascular, they receive nutrition from the substances that diffuse through the blood vessels of the underlying connective tissue. **Glands** are structures that are made up of epithelial tissue and are involved in secretion of fluids. They synthesize substances, such as hormones, and then release them into the bloodstream, into inner-body cavities, or onto the surface of the body. Epithelial tissue has five main functions: (1) to protect underlying tissue from toxins and physical trauma, (2) to absorb substances in the digestive tract lining, (3) to regulate and excrete chemicals between body cavities and underlying tissue surfaces, (4) to secrete hormones into the blood vascular system, and (5) to detect sensations.

Connective tissue fills internal spaces and is never exposed to the outside of the body. It provides structural support for the body and stores energy. This type of tissue is also a protective barrier for delicate organs and for the body against microorganisms. Connective tissue is made up of cells, ground substance, and fibers. The cells are surrounded by extracellular fluid. The ground substance is a viscous substance that is clear and colorless and contains glycosaminoglycans and proteoglycans to keep the collagen fibers within the intercellular spaces. The fibers can be collagenous, which bind bones to other tissues; elastic, which allow organs to stretch and return to their original form; or reticular, which form a scaffolding for other cells. Connective tissue can be described as loose or dense based on how many cells are present and how tightly the fibers are woven together in the tissue.

Muscle tissue has characteristics that make it specialized for contraction, which is the force that produces movement in the body. It also helps the body maintain posture and is responsible for controlling body temperature. Three types of muscle tissue are found in the human body: skeletal, smooth, and cardiac. **Skeletal muscle** contracts voluntarily according to impulses of the central nervous system. It helps support the body and maintain its posture. It also carries out movements of the body. Smooth and cardiac muscle tissue contract involuntarily. They work without conscious thought or impulse to regulate bodily functions. **Smooth muscle** is found in blood vessels and hollow organs, such as the urinary bladder. **Cardiac muscle** is found solely in the heart.

Neural tissue conducts electrical impulses, which help send information and instructions throughout the body. Most of it is concentrated in the brain and spinal cord. Neural tissue comprises neurons and neuroglia. The **neurons** receive and transmit impulses, while the **neuroglia** provide nutrients to the neuron and help pass the impulses from the neurons through the tissue.

Three Primary Body Planes
Since humans can take on many different positions, it is important to learn about the body from a standard position. Directional and regional descriptions refer to the body in a standard anatomical position, which is the body standing with lower limbs together with feet flat on the floor and facing forward, arms at the sides with palms facing forward and thumbs pointing away from the body, and head and eyes facing forward. This standard position avoids confusion when discussing the body and making comparisons between individuals.

Body planes are the hypothetical geometric planes that divide the body into different sections. There are three primary planes of the body. The **transverse plane** is a horizontal plane that separates the superior, or top, portion of the body from the inferior, or bottom, portion of the body. It is parallel to the ground and runs through the center of the body. The **sagittal plane** is a vertical plane that separates the right and left portions of the body. It runs perpendicular to the ground. The **midsagittal plane** runs through the center of the body, splitting the head into two equal parts, and all other sagittal planes are parallel to it. The **coronal plane** is a vertical plane that separates the anterior, or front, and posterior, or back, portions of the body. The planes of the body can be used to identify the location of an individual's organs and to describe anatomical motion. The three main planes of the body create an X-Y-Z coordinate system to describe the motion in a three-dimensional manner. The planes are also helpful for describing embryologic changes and development. When a human embryo first develops, the coronal plane of the embryo is horizontal, or parallel to the ground in standard anatomical position of the mother. As the embryo develops into a fetus, its position changes within the mother, and the coronal plane becomes vertical, or perpendicular to the ground with the mother in standard anatomical position.

Medical imaging technology makes use of the body planes. Ultrasounds, CT scans, MRI scans, and PET scans allow images of the body to be seen in all three dimensions. This allows medical issues and the location of anatomical anomalies to be pinpointed within the body.

Body Planes

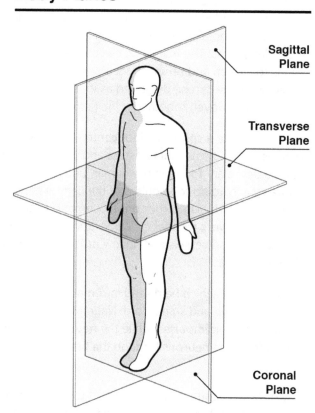

Terms of Direction

In addition to the body planes, using consistent directional terms aids in understanding the human body. It allows different structures to be compared to each other within the same body. There are two other body positions that can be studied in addition to the anatomical position. The **supine** position is when an individual is lying down, face up, in the anatomical position. The **prone** position is when an individual is lying down, face down, in the anatomical position.

There are distinct directional terms used to study the human body. The terms each have an equal and opposite term to describe the opposite side or opposing view of the body. **Anterior** means at or near the front of the body. **Posterior** means at or near the back of the body. The **midline** is the imaginary vertical line that splits the body into equal parts on the left and right. **Lateral** means farther from the midline. **Medial** means closer to the midline. **Superior** means toward the upper part of a structure or toward the head. **Inferior** means toward the lower part of a structure or away from the head. **Superficial** indicates that something is close to the surface of the body. **Deep** means away from the surface of the body. **Proximal** describes something as being near the origin of a structure, whereas **distal** describes it as being away from the origin of a structure. Most of these terms can also be used in combination. For example, a view of the front of the body from above could be called an **anterosuperior** view.

Body Regions

Body regions help separate the body into distinct anatomical compartments. The **axial** part of the body includes everything around the center of the body except the limbs. The **appendicular** part of the body comprises the appendages or limbs. The following table contains a list of body region terms and which part of the body they refer to.

Term	Body Region
Axial	
Head and Neck	
Cephalic	Head
Cervical	Neck
Cranial	Skull
Frontal	Forehead
Nasal	Nose
Occipital	Base of skull
Oral	Mouth
Ocular	Eyes
Thorax	
Axillary	Armpit
Costal	Ribs
Deltoid	Shoulder
Mammary	Breast
Pectoral	Chest
Scapular	Shoulder blade
Sternal	Breastbone
Vertebral	Backbone
Abdomen	
Abdominal	Abdomen
Gluteal	Buttocks
Inguinal	Bend of hip
Lumbar	Lower back
Pelvic	Area between hip bones
Perineal	Area between anus and external genitalia
Pubic	Genitals
Sacral	End of vertebral column
Appendicular	
Upper Extremity	
Antebrachial	Forearm
Antecubital	Inner elbow
Brachial	Upper arm
Carpal	Wrist
Cubital	Elbow
Digital	Fingers and toes
Manual	Hand
Palmar	Palm

Lower Extremity	
Crural	Shin
Femoral	Thigh
Patellar	Front of knee
Pedal	Foot
Plantar	Arch of foot
Popliteal	Back of knee
Sural	Calf
Tarsal	Ankle

Abdominopelvic Regions and Quadrants

The abdominopelvic region of the body can be divided into four quadrants and nine regions. These areas are used to divide the region into smaller areas, since there are quite a few organs and structures located within the abdomen. The four quadrants are created by intersecting a sagittal plane with a transverse plane through the navel. These quadrants are often used by clinicians to pinpoint where abdominal pain is originating. It is important to note that the directional terms that are used refer to that location on the person's body and are not from the clinician's point of view. For example, when looking at a picture of the abdomen, the right upper quadrant is on the left side of the picture when the body is facing forward. The **right upper quadrant** contains the right kidney, a small portion of the stomach, the duodenum, the gallbladder, the head of the pancreas, the right portion of the liver, parts of the small intestine, and parts of the transverse and ascending colon. Pain in this region is often caused by gallbladder inflammation, liver inflammation, or stomach ulcers.

The **left upper quadrant** contains the left kidney, the left portion of the liver, part of the stomach, the spleen, the pancreas, portions of the transvers and descending colon, and parts of the small intestine. Pain in this region is often caused by abnormal rotations of the intestine and colon. The **right lower quadrant** contains the cecum, appendix, part of the small intestine, the right ureter, and the right half of the female reproductive system. Appendicitis pain is associated with this quadrant. The **left lower quadrant** contains most of the small intestine, some of the large intestine, the left ureter, and the left half of the female reproductive system. Pelvic inflammatory disease, ovarian cysts, and inflammation of the large intestine can cause pain in this region.

The nine regions of the abdomen are created by two parasagittal planes and two transverse planes centered around the navel. Once again, the directional terms associated with these regions are from the point of view of the individual's body and not the clinician's view. The nine divisions are the right hypochondriac, left hypochondriac, epigastric, right lumbar, left lumbar, umbilical, right iliac, left iliac, and hypogastric. The **perineum** is the area below the hypogastric region, at the bottom of the abdominopelvic cavity, and can sometimes be considered a tenth region. Most organs are located within two or more regions. The **right hypochondriac region** contains parts of the gallbladder, the right kidney, the small intestine, and the liver. The **left hypochondriac** region contains parts of the left kidney, the pancreas, the stomach, the spleen, and the colon.

The **epigastric region** contains the adrenal glands, most of the stomach, and parts of the liver, pancreas, duodenum, and spleen. The **right lumbar region** contains parts of the gallbladder, the left kidney, the liver, and the ascending colon. The **left lumbar region** contains parts of the descending colon, the left kidney, and the spleen. The **umbilical region** contains the navel and parts of the small intestine, both kidneys, and the transverse colon. The **right iliac region** contains the appendix, cecum, and right iliac fossa. The **left iliac region** contains parts of the descending colon, the sigmoid colon, and the left iliac fossa. The **hypogastric region** contains the organs around the pubic bone, including the bladder, the anus, organs of the reproductive system, and part of the sigmoid colon.

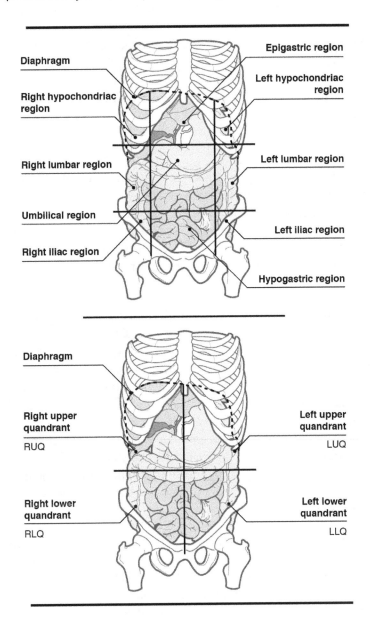

Cell Structure and Function

Although there are trillions of cells in the human body, there are only two hundred different types of cells. The **cell** is the basic functional unit of all living organisms. Humans are made up of eukaryotic cells, which means that the cells contain their DNA in a nucleus that is bound by a membrane, and the cells contain organelles. Organelles are membrane-enclosed structures that each have a specific function. The outside of each cell is surrounded by a phospholipid bilayer membrane, which means that it is a two-layer membrane made up of a chain of phospholipid molecules. Phospholipids have a hydrophobic tail and a hydrophilic head, so the tails of the two layers face each other on the inside, and the hydrophilic heads face the extracellular and internal cellular environments. Molecules can pass through the membrane in a regulated manner. The nucleus of the cell also has a membrane around it to protect the delicate and important DNA inside. The DNA of each cell contains important genetic information from the parent cells and to be passed down to daughter cells. Each organelle contributes a different function to the cell. The endoplasmic reticulum is a network of membranous sacs and tubes that are responsible for packaging and transporting proteins into vesicles to move them out of the cell. The flagella are clusters of microtubules that stick out of the plasma membrane and help the cell move around. The peroxisome contains enzymes that are involved in the cell's metabolic functions. The mitochondrion is the most important cell organelle, as it is responsible for generating the cell's ATP by aerobic cellular respiration. Lysosomes are responsible for digestion of macromolecules. The Golgi apparatus is responsible for composition, modification, organization, and secretion of cell products. Ribosomes make up a complex that manufactures proteins within the cell.

Respiratory System

The **respiratory system** is responsible for gas exchange between air and the blood, mainly via the act of breathing. It is divided into two sections: the upper respiratory system and the lower respiratory system. The **upper respiratory system** consists of the nose, the nasal cavity and sinuses, and the pharynx, while the **lower respiratory system** comprises the larynx (voice box), the trachea (windpipe), the small passageways leading to the lungs, and the lungs. The upper respiratory system is responsible for filtering, warming, and humidifying the air that gets passed to the lower respiratory system, protecting the lower respiratory system's more delicate tissue surfaces.

The human body has two lungs, each having its own distinct characteristics. The right lung is divided into three lobes (superior, middle, and inferior), and the left lung is divided into two lobes (superior and inferior). The left lung is smaller than the right lung, most likely because it shares space in the chest cavity with the heart. Together, the lungs contain approximately fifteen hundred miles of airway passages, which are the site of gas exchange during the act of breathing. When a breath of air is inhaled, oxygen enters the nose or mouth and passes into the sinuses, which is where the temperature and humidity of the air get regulated. The air then passes into the trachea and is filtered. From there, it travels into the bronchi and reaches the lungs. Bronchi are lined with cilia and mucus that collect dust and germs along the way. Within the lungs, oxygen and carbon dioxide are exchanged between the air in the **alveoli,** a type of airway passage in the lungs, and the blood in the **pulmonary capillaries**, a type of blood vessel in the lungs. Oxygen-rich blood returns to the heart and gets pumped through the systemic circuit. Carbon dioxide-rich air is exhaled from the body.

The respiratory system has many important functions in the body. Primarily, it is responsible for **pulmonary ventilation**, or the process of breathing. During pulmonary ventilation, air is inhaled through the nasal cavity or oral cavity and then moves through the pharynx, larynx, and trachea before reaching the lungs. Air is exhaled following the same pathway. When air is inhaled, the diaphragm and external intercostal muscles contract, causing the rib cage to rise and the volume of the lungs to increase. When air is exhaled, the muscles relax, and the volume of the lungs decreases. The respiratory system also provides a large area for gas exchange between the air and the circulating blood. During the process of external respiration, oxygen and carbon dioxide are exchanged within the lungs. Oxygen goes into the bloodstream, binds to hemoglobin in the red blood cells, and circulates through the body. Carbon dioxide moves from the deoxygenated blood into the alveoli of the lungs and is then exhaled from the body through the nose or mouth. Internal respiration is a process that allows gases to be exchanged between the circulating blood and body tissues. Arteries carry oxygenated blood throughout the body. When the oxygenated blood reaches narrow capillaries in the body tissue, the red blood cells release the oxygen.

The oxygen then diffuses through the capillary walls into the body tissues. At the same time, carbon dioxide diffuses from the body tissues into the blood of the narrow capillaries. Veins carry the deoxygenated blood back to the lungs for waste removal. Another function of the respiratory system is that it produces the sounds that the body makes for speaking and singing, as well as for nonverbal communication. The larynx is also known as the voice box. When air is exhaled, it passes through the larynx. The muscles of the larynx move the arytenoid cartilages, which then push the vocal cords together. When air passes through the larynx while the vocal cords are being pushed together, the vocal cords vibrate and create sound. Higher-pitched sounds are made when the vocal cords are vibrating more rapidly, and lower-pitched sounds are made when the vibrations are slower. The respiratory system also helps with an individual's sense of smell. Olfactory fibers line the nasal cavity. When air enters the nose, chemicals within the air bind to the olfactory fibers. Neurons then take the olfactory signal from the nasal cavity to the olfactory area of the brain for sensory processing. In addition to these major functions, the respiratory system also protects the delicate respiratory surfaces from environmental variations and defends them against pathogens and helps regulate blood volume, blood pressure, and body fluid pH.

Respiratory System

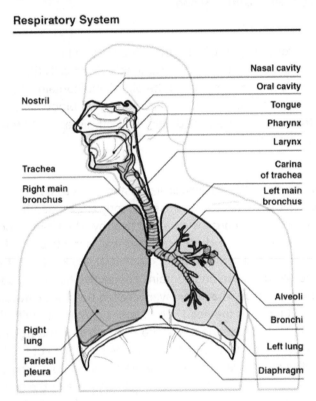

Infections of the respiratory system are common. Most upper respiratory infections are caused by viruses and include the common cold and sinusitis. Bacterial infections of the upper respiratory system are less common and include epiglottitis and croup. This part of the respiratory system gets infected by an organism entering the nasal or oral cavity and invading the mucosa that is present. The organism then begins to destroy the epithelium of the upper respiratory system. Infections of the lower respiratory system can be caused by viruses or bacteria. They include bronchitis, bronchiolitis, and pneumonia. These infections are caused by an organism entering the airway and multiplying itself in or on the epithelium in the lower respiratory system. Inflammation ensues, as well as increased mucus secretion and impaired function of the cilia lining the airways and lungs.

Cardiovascular System

The **cardiovascular system** is composed of the heart and blood vessels. It has three main functions in the human body. First, it transports nutrients, oxygen, and hormones through the blood to the body tissues and cells that need them. It also helps to remove metabolic waste, such as carbon dioxide and nitrogenous waste, through the bloodstream. Second, the cardiovascular system protects the body from attack by foreign microorganisms and toxins. The white blood cells, antibodies, and complement proteins that circulate within the blood help defend the body against these pathogens. The clotting system of the blood also helps protect the body from infection when there is blood loss following an injury. Lastly, this system helps regulate body temperature, fluid pH, and water content of the cells.

Blood Vessels

Blood circulates throughout the body in vessels called arteries, veins, and capillaries. These vessels are muscular tubes that allow gas exchange to occur. **Arteries** carry oxygen-rich blood from the heart to the other tissues of the body. **Veins** collect oxygen-depleted blood from tissues and organs and return it back to the heart. **Capillaries** are the smallest of the blood vessels and do not function individually; instead, they work together in a unit called a **capillary bed**.

Blood

Blood is an important vehicle for transport of oxygen, nutrients, and hormones throughout the body. It is composed of plasma and formed elements, which include red blood cells (RBCs), white blood cells (WBCs), and platelets. **Plasma** is the liquid matrix of the blood and contains dissolved proteins. *RBCs* contain **hemoglobin**, which carries oxygen through the blood. Red blood cells also transport carbon dioxide. **WBCs** are part of the immune system and help fight off diseases. **Platelets** contain enzymes and other factors that help with blood clotting.

Heart

The heart, which is the main organ of the cardiovascular system, acts as a pump and circulates blood throughout the body. Gases, nutrients, and waste are constantly exchanged between the circulating blood and interstitial fluid, keeping tissues and organs alive and healthy. The heart is located behind the sternum, on the left side, in the front of the chest. The heart wall is made up of three distinct layers. The outer layer, called the **epicardium,** is a serous membrane that is also known as the **visceral pericardium**. The middle layer is called the **myocardium** and contains connective tissue, blood vessels, and nerves within its layers of cardiac muscle tissue. The inner layer is called the **endocardium,** and is made up of a simple squamous epithelium. It includes the heart valves and is continuous with the endothelium of the attached blood vessels. The heart has four chambers: the **right atrium**, the **right ventricle,** the **left atrium,** and the **left ventricle**. The atrium and ventricle on the same side of the heart have an opening between them that is regulated by a valve. The valve maintains blood flow in only one direction, moving from the atrium to the ventricle, and prevents backflow. The right side of the heart has a **tricuspid valve** (because it has three leaflets) between the chambers, and the left side of the heart has a **bicuspid valve** (with two leaflets) between the chambers, also called the **mitral valve**. Oxygen-poor blood from the body enters the right atrium through the superior vena cava and the inferior vena cava and is pumped into the right ventricle. The blood then enters the pulmonary trunk and flows into the pulmonary arteries, where it can become re-oxygenated. Oxygen-rich blood from the lungs then flows into the left atrium from four pulmonary veins, passes into the left ventricle, enters the aorta, and gets pumped to the rest of the body.

Cardiac Cycle

The **cardiac cycle** is the series of events that occur when the heart beats. During the cardiac cycle, blood is circulated throughout the pulmonary and systemic circuits of the body. There are two phases of the cardiac cycle—diastole and systole. During the **diastole** period, the ventricles of the heart are relaxed and are not contracting. Blood is flowing passively from the left atrium to the left ventricle and from the right atrium to the right ventricle through the atrioventricular valves. At the end of the diastole phase, both the left and right atria contract, and an additional amount of blood is pushed through to the respective ventricles. The **systole** period occurs when the left and right ventricles both contract. The aortic valve opens at the left ventricle and pushes blood through to the aorta, and the pulmonary valve opens at the right ventricle and pushes blood through to the pulmonary artery. During this phase, the atrioventricular valves are closed, and blood does not enter the ventricles from the atria.

Types of Circulation

Circulating blood carries oxygen, nutrients, and hormones throughout the body, which are vital for sustaining life. There are two types of cardiac circulation: pulmonary circulation and systemic circulation. The heart is responsible for pumping blood in both types of circulation. The **pulmonary circulatory system** carries blood between the heart and the lungs. It works in conjunction with the respiratory system to facilitate external respiration. Deoxygenated blood flows to the lungs through the vessels of the cardiovascular system to obtain oxygen and release carbon dioxide from the respiratory system. Blood that is rich with oxygen flows from the lungs back to the heart. Pulmonary circulation occurs only in the pulmonary loop. The pulmonary trunk takes the deoxygenated blood from the right ventricle to the arterioles and capillary beds of the lungs. Once the blood that is filling these spaces has been reoxygenated, it passes into the pulmonary veins and is transported to the left atrium of the heart. The **systemic circulatory system** carries blood from the heart to the rest of the body and works in conjunction with the respiratory system to facilitate internal respiration. The oxygenated blood flows out of the heart through the vessels and reaches the body tissues, while the deoxygenated blood flows through the vessels from the body back to the heart. Unlike the pulmonary loop, the systemic loop covers the whole body. Oxygen-rich blood moves out of the left ventricle into the aorta. The aorta circulates the blood to the systemic arteries and then to the arterioles and capillary beds that are present in the body tissues, where oxygen and nutrients are released into the tissues. The deoxygenated blood then moves from the capillary beds to the venules and systemic veins. The systemic veins bring the blood back to the right atrium of the heart.

Here's a visual representation of this:

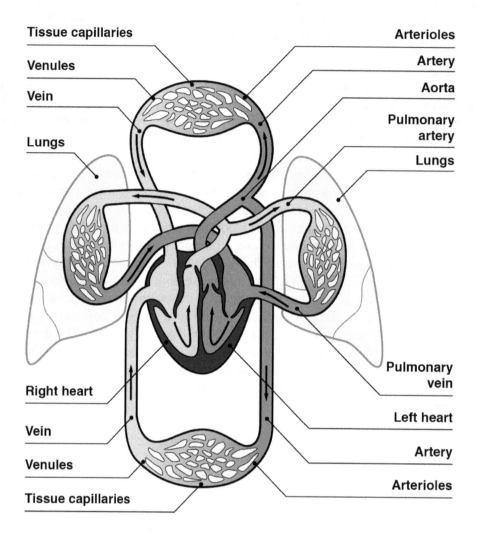

Gastrointestinal System

The **gastrointestinal system** is a group of organs that work together to fuel the body by transforming food and liquids into energy. After food is ingested, it passes through the **alimentary canal**, or **GI tract,** which comprises the mouth, pharynx, esophagus, stomach, small intestine, and large intestine. Each organ has a specific function to aid in digestion. Listed below are seven steps that incorporate the transformation of food as it travels through the gastrointestinal system.

- Ingestion: Food and liquids enter the alimentary canal through the mouth.

- Mechanical processing: Food is torn up by the teeth and swirled around by the tongue to facilitate swallowing.

- Digestion: Chemicals and enzymes break down complex molecules, such as sugars, lipids, and proteins, into smaller molecules that can be absorbed by the digestive epithelium.

- Secretion: Most of the acids, buffers, and enzymes that aid in digestion are secreted by the accessory organs, but some are provided by the digestive tract.

- Absorption: Vitamins, electrolytes, organic molecules, and water are absorbed by the digestive epithelium and moved to the interstitial fluid of the digestive tract.

- Compaction: Indigestible materials and organic wastes are dehydrated and compacted before elimination from the body.

- Excretion: Waste products are secreted into the digestive tract.

Mouth and Stomach

The mouth is the first point at which food and drink enter the gastrointestinal system. It is where food is chewed and torn apart by the teeth. Salivary glands in the mouth produce saliva, which is used to break down starches. The tongue also helps grip the food as it is being chewed and push it posteriorly toward the esophagus. The food and drink then move down the esophagus by the process of swallowing and into the stomach. The inferior end of the esophagus, at the stomach end, has a lower esophageal sphincter that closes off the esophagus and traps food in the stomach. The stomach stores food so that the body has time to digest large meals. It secretes enzymes and acids and also helps with mechanical processing through **peristalsis** or muscular contractions. The upper muscle of the stomach relaxes to let food in, and the lower muscle mixes the food with the digestive juices. The stomach secretes stomach acid to help break down proteins. Once digestion is completed in the stomach, the broken-down contents, called **chyme,** are passed into the small intestine.

Small Intestine

The **small intestine** is a thin tube that is approximately ten feet long and takes up most of the space in the abdominal cavity. The three structural parts of the small intestine are the duodenum, the jejunum, and the ileum. The **duodenum** is shaped like a C and receives the chyme from the stomach along with the digestive juices from the pancreas and the liver. The jejunum is the middle portion of the small intestine. It is the section with the most circular folds and villi to increase its surface area. The digestive products are absorbed into the bloodstream in the jejunum. The ileum follows the jejunum portion of the small intestine. It mainly absorbs bile acids and vitamin B12 and passes it into the bloodstream. The ileum connects to the large intestine. The entire small intestine secretes enzymes and has folds that increase its surface area and allow for maximum absorption of nutrients from the digested food. The small intestine digestive juice along with juices from the pancreas to liver in combination with peristalsis work to complete the digestion of starches, proteins, and carbohydrates. By the time food leaves the small intestine, approximately 90 percent of the nutrients have been absorbed. These nutrients are carried to the rest of the body. The undigested and unabsorbed food particles are passed into the large intestine.

Large Intestine

The **large intestine** is a long, thick tube that is about five feet in length, also known as the **colon.** It is the final part of the gastrointestinal tract. It has five main sections. The ascending colon connects to the small intestine and runs upward along the right side of the body. It also includes the appendix. The transverse colon runs parallel to the ground from the ascending colon to the left side of the abdominal cavity. The descending colon runs downward along the left side of the body. The sigmoid colon is an S-shaped region that connects the descending colon to the rectum. The rectum is the end of the colon and is a temporary storage place for feces. The function of the large intestine is to absorb water from the digested food and transport waste to be excreted from the body. It also contains symbiotic bacteria that break down the waste products even further, allowing for any additional nutrients to be absorbed. The final waste products are converted to stool and then stored in the rectum.

Pancreas

The pancreas is a large gland that is about 6 inches long. It secretes buffers and digestive enzymes into the duodenum of the small intestine. It contains specific enzymes for each type of food molecule, such as amylases for carbohydrates, lipases for lipids, and proteases for proteins. This digestive function of the pancreas is called the exocrine role of the pancreas. The cells of the pancreas are present in clusters called **acini**. The digestive enzymes are secreted into the middle of the acini into intralobular ducts. These ducts drain into the main pancreatic duct, which then drains into the duodenum.

In addition to these main organs, the gastrointestinal system has a few accessory organs that help break down food without having the food or liquid pass directly through them. The liver produces and secretes **bile,** which is important for the digestion of lipids. The bile mixes with the fat in food and helps dissolve it into the water contents within the small intestine, which helps fatty foods to be digested. The liver also plays a large role in the regulation of circulating levels of carbohydrates, amino acids, and lipids in the body. Excess nutrients are removed by the liver and deficiencies are corrected with its stored nutrients. The gallbladder is responsible for storing and concentrating bile before it gets secreted into the small intestine. It recycles the bile from the small intestine so that it can be used to digest subsequent meals.

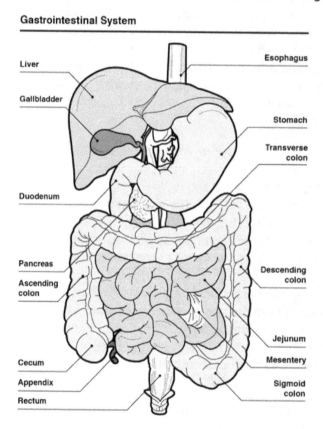

Gastrointestinal System

Neuromuscular System

The **neuromuscular system** is composed of all of the muscles in the human body and the nerves that control them. Every movement that the body makes is controlled by the brain. The nervous system and the muscular system work together to link thoughts and actions. Neurons from the nervous system can relay information from the brain to muscle tissue so fast that an individual does not even realize it is happening. Some body movements and functions are voluntary, but others are involuntary, such as the heart beating and the lungs breathing.

Nervous System

The nervous system is made up of the central nervous system (CNS) and the peripheral nervous system (PNS). The CNS includes the brain and the spinal cord, while the PNS includes the rest of the neural tissue that is not included in the CNS. **Neurons,** or nerve cells, are the main cells responsible for transferring and processing information between the brain and other parts of the body. **Neuroglia** are cells that support the neurons by providing a framework around them and isolating them from the surrounding environment.

Central Nervous System

The CNS is located within the dorsal body cavity, with the brain in the cranial cavity and the spinal cord in the spinal canal. The brain is protected by the skull, and the spinal cord is protected by the vertebrae. The brain is made up of white and gray matter. The white matter contains axons and oligodendrocytes. **Axons** are the long projection ends of neurons that are responsible for transmitting signals through the nervous system, while **oligodendrocytes** act as insulators for the axons and provide support for them. The gray matter consists of neurons and fibers that are unmyelinated. Neurons are nerve cells that receive and transmit information through electrical and chemical signals. Glial cells and astrocytes are located in both types of tissue. Different types of glial cells have different roles in the CNS. Some are immunoprotective, while others provide a scaffolding for other types of nerve cells. **Astrocytes** provide nutrients to neurons and clear out metabolites. The spinal cord has projections within it from the PNS. This allows the information that is received from the areas of the body that the PNS reaches to be transmitted to the brain. The CNS as a whole is responsible for processing and coordinating sensory data and motor commands. It receives information from all parts of the body, processes it, and then sends out action commands in response. Some of the reactions are conscious, while others are unconscious.

Infections of the CNS include **encephalitis**, which is an inflammation of the brain, and **poliomyelitis**, which is caused by a virus and causes muscle weakness. Other developmental neurological disorders include ADHD and autism. Some diseases of the CNS can occur later in life and affect the aging brain, such as Alzheimer's disease and Parkinson's disease. Cancers that occur in the CNS can be very serious and have high mortality rates.

Peripheral Nervous System

The PNS consists of the nerves and ganglia that are located within the body outside of the brain and spinal cord. It connects the rest of the body, organs, and limbs to the CNS. Unlike the CNS, the PNS does not have any bony structures protecting it. The PNS is responsible for relaying sensory information and motor commands between the CNS and peripheral tissues and systems. It has two subdivisions, known as the afferent, or sensory, and efferent, or motor, divisions. The **afferent division** relays sensory information to the CNS and supplies information from the skin and joints about the body's sensation and balance. It carries information away from the stimulus back to the brain. The afferent division provides the brain with sensory information about things such as taste, smell, and vision. It also monitors organs, vessels, and glands for changes in activity and can alert the brain to send out appropriate responses for bringing the body back to homeostasis. The **efferent division** transmits motor commands to muscles and glands. It sends information from the CNS to the organs and muscles to provide appropriate responses to sensations. The electrical responses from the neurons are initiated in the CNS, but the axons terminate in the organs that are part of the PNS. The efferent division consists of the **autonomic nervous system (ANS),** which regulates activity of smooth muscle, cardiac muscle, and glands, and allows the brain to control heart rate, blood pressure, and body temperature, and the **somatic nervous system (SNS),** which controls skeletal muscle contractions and allows the brain to control body movement.

Diseases of the PNS can affect single nerves or the whole system. Single nerve damage, or **mononeuropathy,** can occur when a nerve gets compressed due to trauma or a tumor. It can also be damaged as a result of being trapped under another part of the body that is increasing in size, such as in carpal tunnel syndrome. These diseases can cause pain and numbness at the affected area.

Autonomic Nervous System

The **autonomic nervous system** is made up of pathways that extend from the CNS to the organs, muscles, and glands of the body. The pathway is made up of two separate neurons. The first neuron has a cell body that is located within the CNS, for example, within the spinal cord. The axon of that first neuron synapses with the cell body of the second neuron. Part of the second neuron innervates the organ, muscle, or gland that the pathway is responsible for.

The autonomic nervous system consists of the sympathetic nervous system and the parasympathetic nervous system. The **sympathetic nervous system** is activated when mentally stressful or physically dangerous situations are faced, also known as "fight or flight" situations. Neurotransmitters are released that increase heart rate and blood flow in critical areas, such as the muscles, and decrease activity for nonessential functions, such as digestion. This system is activated unconsciously. The **parasympathetic system** has some voluntary control. It releases neurotransmitters that allow the body to function in a restful state. Heart rate and other sympathetic responses are often decreased when the parasympathetic system is activated.

Somatic Nervous System and the Reflex Arc

The **somatic nervous system** is considered the voluntary part of the PNS. It comprises motor neurons whose axons innervate skeletal muscle. However, nerve muscles and muscle cells do not come into direct contact with each other. Instead, the neurotransmitter acetylcholine transfers the signal between the nerve cell and muscle cell. These junctions are called **neuromuscular junctions**. When the muscle cell receives the signal from the nerve cell, it causes the muscle to contract.

Although most muscle contractions are voluntary, reflexes are a type of muscle contraction that is involuntary. A **reflex** is an instantaneous movement that occurs in response to a stimulus and is controlled by a neural pathway called a **reflex arc.** The reflex arc carries the sensory information from the receptor to the spinal cord and then carries the response back to the muscles. Many sensory neurons synapse in the spinal cord so that reflex actions can occur faster, without waiting for the signal to travel to the brain and back. For somatic reflexes, stimuli activate somatic receptors in the skin, muscles, and tendons. Then, afferent nerve fibers carry signals from the receptors to the spinal cord or brain stem. The signal reaches an integrating center, which is where the neurons synapse within the spinal cord or brain stem. Efferent nerve fibers then carry motor nerve signals to the muscles, and the muscles carry out the response.

Muscular System

There are approximately seven hundred muscles in the body. They are attached to the bones of the skeletal system and make up half of the body's weight. There are three types of muscle tissue in the body: skeletal muscle, smooth muscle, and cardiac muscle. An important characteristic of all types of muscle is that they are **excitable,** which means that they respond to electrical stimuli.

Skeletal Muscles

Skeletal muscle tissue is a voluntary, striated muscle tissue, which means that the contractile fibers of the tissue are aligned parallel so that they appear to form stripes when viewed under a microscope. Most skeletal muscle are attached to bones by intermediary tendons. Tendons are bundles of collagen fibers.

When nerve cells release acetylcholine at the neuromuscular junction, skeletal muscle contracts. The skeletal muscle tissue then pulls on the bones of the skeleton and causes body movement.

Smooth Muscles

Smooth muscle tissue is an involuntary nonstriated muscle tissue. It has greater elasticity than striated muscle but still maintains its contractile ability. Smooth muscle tissue can be of the single-unit variety or the multi-unit variety. Most smooth muscle tissues are single unit where the cells all act in unison and the whole muscle contracts or relaxes. Single-unit smooth muscle lines the blood vessels, urinary tract, and digestive tract. It helps to move fluids and solids along the digestive tract, allows for expansion of the urinary bladder as it fills and helps move blood through the vessels. Multi-unit smooth muscle is found in the iris of the eye, large elastic arteries, and the trachea.

Cardiac Muscles

Cardiac muscle tissue is an involuntary striated muscle that is only found in the walls of the heart. The cells that make up the tissue contract together to pump blood through the veins and arteries. This tissue has high contractility and extreme endurance, since it pumps for an individual's entire lifetime without any rest. Each cardiac muscle cell has finger-like projections, called **intercalated disks**, at each end that overlap with the same projections on neighboring cells. The intercalated disks form tight junctions between the cells so that they do not separate as the heart beats and so that electrochemical signals are passed from cell to cell quickly and efficiently.

Reproductive System

The **reproductive system** is responsible for producing, storing, nourishing, and transporting functional reproductive cells, or **gametes**, in the human body. It includes the reproductive organs, also known as **gonads,** the reproductive tract, the accessory glands and organs that secrete fluids into the reproductive tract, and the **perineal structures**, which are the external genitalia. The human male and female reproductive systems are very different from each other.

The male gonads are called **testes.** The testes secrete androgens, mainly testosterone, and produce and store one-half billion **sperms cells**, which are the male gametes, each day. An **androgen** is a steroid hormone that controls the development and maintenance of male characteristics. Once the sperm are mature, they move through a duct system where they are mixed with additional fluids that are secreted by accessory glands, forming a mixture called **semen.** The sperm cells in semen are responsible for fertilization of the female gametes to produce offspring. The male reproductive system has a few accessory organs as well, which are located inside the body. The **prostate gland** and the **seminal vesicles** provide additional fluid that serves as nourishment to the sperm during ejaculation. The **vas deferens** is responsible for transportation of sperm to the urethra. The **bulbourethral glands** produce a lubricating fluid for the urethra that also neutralizes the residual acidity left behind by urine.

The female gonads are called **ovaries.** Ovaries generally produce one immature gamete, or **oocyte,** per month. The ovaries are also responsible for secreting the hormones estrogen and progesterone. When the oocyte is released from the ovary, it travels along the uterine tubes, or **Fallopian tubes**, and then into the **uterus.** The uterus opens into the vagina. When sperm cells enter the vagina, they swim through the uterus. If they fertilize the oocyte, they do so in the Fallopian tubes. The resulting zygote travels down the tube and implants into the uterine wall. The uterus protects and nourishes the developing embryo for nine months until it is ready for the outside environment. If the oocyte is not fertilized, it is released in the uterine, or menstrual, cycle. The **menstrual cycle** usually occurs monthly and involves the shedding of the functional part of the uterine lining. **Mammary glands** are a specialized accessory organ of the female reproductive system. The mammary glands are located in the breast tissue of females. During pregnancy, the glands begin to grow as the cells proliferate in preparation for lactation. After pregnancy, the cells begin to secrete nutrient-filled milk, which is transferred into a duct system and out through the nipple for nourishment of the baby.

Integumentary System

The **integumentary system** protects the body from damage from the outside. It consists of skin and its appendages, including hair, nails, and sweat glands. This system functions as a cushion, a waterproof layer, a temperature regulator, and a protectant of the deeper tissues within the body. It also excretes waste from the body. The skin is the largest organ of the human body, consisting of two layers called the epidermis and the dermis. The **epidermis** can be classified as thick or thin. Most of the body is covered with thin skin but areas such as the palm of the hands are covered with thick skin. The epidermis is responsible for synthesizing vitamin D when exposed to UV rays. Vitamin D is essential to the body for the processes of calcium and phosphorus absorption, which maintain healthy bones. The **dermis** lies under the epidermis and consists of a superficial papillary layer and a deeper reticular layer. The **papillary layer** is made up of loose connective tissue and contains capillaries and the axons of sensory neurons. The **reticular layer** is a meshwork of tightly packed irregular connective tissue and contains blood vessels, hair follicles, nerves, sweat glands, and sebaceous glands.

The three major functions of skin are protection, regulation, and sensation. Skin acts as a barrier and protects the body from mechanical impacts, variations in temperature, microorganisms, and chemicals. It regulates body temperature, peripheral circulation, and fluid balance by secreting sweat. It also contains a large network of nerve cells that relay changes in the external environment to the body.

Hair provides many functions for the human body. It provides sensation, protects against heat loss, and filters air that is taken in through the nose. Nails provide a hard layer of protection over soft skin. Sweat glands and sebaceous glands are two important exocrine glands found in the skin. **Sweat glands** regulate temperature and remove bodily waste by secreting water, nitrogenous waste, and sodium salts to the surface of the body. **Sebaceous glands** secrete **sebum,** which is an oily mixture of lipids and proteins. Sebum protects the skin from water loss and bacterial and fungal infections.

Endocrine System

The **endocrine system** is made up of ductless tissues and glands, and is responsible for hormone secretion into either the blood or the interstitial fluid of the human body. **Hormones** are chemical substances that change the metabolic activity of tissues and organs. **Interstitial fluid** is the solution that surrounds tissue cells within the body. This system works closely with the nervous system to regulate the physiological activities of the other systems of the body in order to maintain homeostasis. While the nervous system provides quick, short-term responses to stimuli, the endocrine system acts by releasing hormones into the bloodstream, which then are distributed to the whole body. The response is slow but long lasting, ranging from a few hours to even a few weeks. While regular metabolic reactions are controlled by enzymes, hormones can change the type, activity, or quantity of the enzymes involved in the reaction. They can regulate development and growth, digestive metabolism, mood, and body temperature, among many other things. Often very small amounts of a hormone will lead to large changes in the body.

There are eight major glands in the endocrine system, each with its own specific function. They are described below.

- **Hypothalamus:** This gland is a part of the brain. It connects the nervous system to the endocrine system via the pituitary gland and plays an important role in regulating endocrine organs.

- **Pituitary gland:** This pea-sized gland is found at the bottom of the hypothalamus. It releases hormones that regulate growth, blood pressure, certain functions of the reproductive sex organs, and pain relief, among other things. It also plays an important role in regulating the function of other endocrine glands.

- **Thyroid gland:** This gland releases hormones that are important for metabolism, growth and development, temperature regulation, and brain development during infancy and childhood. Thyroid hormones also monitor the amount of circulating calcium in the body.

- **Parathyroid glands:** These are four pea-sized glands located on the posterior surface of the thyroid. The main hormone that is secreted is called parathyroid hormone (PTH) and helps with the thyroid's regulation of calcium in the body.

- **Thymus gland:** This gland is located in the chest cavity, embedded in connective tissue. It produces several hormones that are important for development and maintenance of normal immunological defenses.

- **Adrenal glands:** One adrenal gland is attached to the top of each kidney. Its major function is to aid in the management of stress.

- **Pancreas:** This gland produces hormones that regulate blood sugar levels in the body.

- **Pineal gland:** The pineal gland secretes the hormone **melatonin**, which can slow the maturation of sperm, oocytes, and reproductive organs. Melatonin also regulates the body's circadian rhythm, which is the natural awake-asleep cycles.

Genitourinary System

The **genitourinary system** encompasses the reproductive organs and the urinary system. They are often grouped together because of their proximity to each other in the body, and, for the male, because of shared pathways. The external male genitalia include the penis, urethra, and scrotum. Both urine and male gametes travel through the urethra within the penis to exit the body. In both the male and female bodies, the urinary system is made up of the kidneys, ureters, urinary bladder, and the urethra. It is the main system responsible for getting rid of the organic waste products, as well as excess water and electrolytes that are generated by the other systems of the body. Regulation of the water and electrolytes also contributes to the maintenance of blood pH.

Under normal circumstances, humans have two functioning **kidneys.** They are the main organs that are responsible for filtering waste products out of the blood and transferring them to urine. Every day, the kidneys filter approximately 120 to 150 quarts of blood and produce one to two quarts of urine. The kidneys are made up of millions of tiny filtering units called **nephrons.** Nephrons have two parts: a **glomerulus,** which is the filter, and a **tubule.** As blood enters the kidneys, the glomerulus allows for fluid and waste products to pass through it and enter the tubule. Blood cells and large molecules, such as proteins, do not pass through and remain in the blood. The filtered fluid and waste then pass through the tubule, where any final essential minerals can be sent back to the bloodstream. The final product at the end of the tubule is called **urine.** The urine travels through the **ureters** into the **urinary bladder**, which is a hollow, elastic muscular organ. As more and more urine enters the urinary bladder, its walls stretch and become thinner so that there is no significant difference in internal pressure. The urinary bladder stores the urine until the body is ready for urination, at which time its muscles contract and force the urine through the urethra and out of the body.

Immune System

The **immune system** comprises cells, tissues, and organs that work together to protect the body. They recognize millions of different microorganisms, such as parasites, bacteria, and fungi, and viruses that can invade and infect the body. When an attack on the body is sensed, immune cells are activated and communicate with each other through an elaborate network. They begin to produce chemicals and recruit other cells to defend the body at the infection site. It is important for the body's immune system to be able to distinguish between pathogens, such as viruses and microorganisms, and the body's own healthy tissue, so that the body does not attack itself. There are two types of immune systems that work to defend the body against infection: the innate system and the adaptive system.

Innate Immune System

The **innate immune system** is triggered when pattern recognition receptors recognize components of microorganisms that are the same among many different varieties, or when damaged or stressed cells send out help signals. It is always primed and ready to fight infections. This system works in a nonspecific way, which means that it works without having a memory of the pathogens it defended against previously and does not provide long-lasting immunity for the body. It does critical work in the first few hours and days of exposure to a pathogen to fight off infection by producing general immune responses, such as by producing inflammation and activating the complement cascade. During inflammation, immune cells that are already present in the injured tissue are activated, and chemicals stimulate inflammation of the tissue to create a physical barrier against the infection. The complement system is a cascade of events that the immune systems starts to help antibodies fight off pathogens. The proteins that are produced first recruit inflammatory cells and then tag the pathogens for destruction by coating them with opsonin. The proteins also put holes in the pathogen's plasma membrane and, lastly, help rid the body of the neutralized invader.

Mechanical, chemical, and surface barriers all function as part of the innate immune system. Mechanical barriers are the first line of defense against pathogens. Both skin and the respiratory tract are examples of mechanical barriers that provide initial protection against infection. The epithelial layer of the skin is an impermeable physical barrier that wards off many infections. When the epithelium sheds, or goes through desquamation, any microbes that are attached to the skin are removed as well. The top layers of skin are also avascular and lack a blood supply, so the environment is not ideal for survival of microbes. The respiratory tract uses a mucociliary escalator to protect against infection. Pathogens get caught in the sticky mucus that lines the respiratory tract and are moved upward toward the throat. If a mechanical barrier is passed and the pathogen enters the body, chemical barriers are activated.

These barriers include cells that have a secondary purpose of fighting off infections. For example, the gastric acid and proteases found in the stomach act as chemical barriers against pathogens that are ingested. They create unfriendly and toxic environments for bacteria to colonize. The group of proteins called **interferons** helps inhibit the replication of viruses. Biological barriers can also help prevent infection. The bacteria that is naturally found in the gastrointestinal tract acts as a biological barrier by creating competition for nutrients and space against pathogenic bacteria. The eyes have a flushing reflex to push out pathogens that may cause infection. Tears are produced by the tear ducts and collect the microbes to be released along with them from the eye.

Adaptive Immune System

The **adaptive immune system** creates a memory of the pathogen that it fought against previously so that the body can respond again in an efficient manner the next time the pathogen is encountered. When **antigens**, or allergens, such as pollen, are encountered, specific antibodies are secreted to inactivate the antigen and protect the body. The response of the adaptive immune system can take several days, which is much longer than the immediate response of the innate immune system. It uses fewer types of cells to produce its immune response compared to the innate immune system as well. The adaptive immune system provides the body with a long-lasting defense mechanism and protection against recurrent infections. Vaccines use the memory of the adaptive immune system to protect individuals against diseases they have never experienced. When vaccines are administered, an active, weakened, or attenuated virus is injected into the body, which mimics the active virus. The adaptive immune system then starts an immune response and creates a memory of the antigens associated with that disease along with the antibodies to fight them off.

Lymphocytes are the specialized cells that are a part of the adaptive immune system. **B cells** and **T cells** are different types of lymphocytes that are derived from multipotent hematopoietic stem cells and that recognize specific target pathogens. B cells are formed in the bone marrow and then move into the lymphatic system and circulate through the body. These cells are called **naive B cells**. Naive B cells express millions of antibodies on their surfaces as well as a B-cell receptor (BCR). The BCR helps with antigen binding, internalization, and processing. It allows the B cell to then initiate signaling pathways and communicate with other immune cells. When a naive B cell encounters an antigen that fits one of its surface antibodies, it begins to mature and differentiates into a memory B cell or a plasma cell. **Memory B cells** retain their surface-bound antibodies. **Plasma cells**, on the other hand, secrete their antibodies instead of keeping them attached to the cell membrane. The freely circulating antibodies can then identify pathogens that are circulating throughout the body.

T cells are also produced in the bone marrow. They then migrate to the thymus where they mature and start to express T-cell receptors (TCRs) as well as one of two other types of receptors—CD4 or CD8. These receptors help T cells identify antigens that are bound to specific receptors on antigen-presenting cells, such as macrophages and dendritic cells. CD4 and CD8 bind to the receptor-antigen complex on these cells, which activates the T cells to produce an immune response. After maturation, the three types of T cells that are produced are helper T cells, cytotoxic T cells, and T regulatory cells. **Helper T cells** express CD4 and help activate B cells, cytotoxic T cells, and other immune cells. **Cytotoxic T cells** express CD8 and remove pathogens and infected host cells. **T regulatory cells** express CD4 and help distinguish between molecules that belong to the individual and foreign molecules.

Malfunctions of the Immune System

An **immunodeficiency** occurs when the body cannot respond to a pathogen because a component of the immune system is inactive. This can be caused by a genetic mutation or by behavior. For example, smoking paralyzes the mucociliary escalator of the respiratory tract, disabling a critical part of the body's innate immune system. If the immune system is not functioning properly, the body may attack its own self and develop an autoimmune disorder. When the body cannot distinguish between itself and foreign pathogens, the immune system becomes overactive and the body attacks itself unnecessarily. To diagnose an autoimmune disease, it is important to identify which antibodies an individual's body is producing and then determine which of those antibodies is attacking the individual itself. Autoantibody tests look for specific antibodies within an individual's tissues; antinuclear antibody tests are specific autoantibody tests that look for antibodies that attack the nuclei of cells; complete blood count tests count the number of red and white cells in the blood, which reveals if the body is actively fighting an infection; and C-reactive protein tests determine whether there is inflammation occurring throughout the body.

Diseases such as type I diabetes and rheumatoid arthritis are autoimmune disorders. The pancreas contains cells that produce insulin to regulate blood sugar levels. In type I diabetes, auto-aggressive T cells infiltrate the pancreas and destroy the insulin-producing beta cells population. Without the insulin-producing cells, the body cannot regulate blood sugar levels on its own and requires external sources of insulin to maintain healthy levels. Rheumatoid arthritis occurs when the body's immune system attacks the joint linings of its own body. This causes inflammation and damage in healthy tissue around the joints, leading to pain and immobility.

Skeletal System

The adult **skeletal system** consists of the 206 bones that make up the skeleton, as well as the cartilage, ligaments, and other connective tissues that stabilize them. Babies are born with roughly three hundred bones, some of which fuse together during growth. Bone is made up of collagen fibers and calcium salts. The calcium salts are strong but brittle, and the collagen fibers are weak but flexible, so the combination makes bone very resistant to shattering.

Axial Skeleton
The **axial skeleton** comprises the bones found in the head, trunk of the body, and vertebrae—a total of eighty bones. It is the central core of the body and is responsible for connecting the pelvis to the rest of the body. The axial skeleton can be divided into the following five parts:

1. The **skull bones** are made up of the cranium and the facial bones. While the skeleton gets frailer with age, the skull remains strong to protect the brain. The cranium is formed from eight flat bones that fit together without spaces in between. These meeting points are called **sutures.** The brain is held in a space inside the cranium called the **cranial vault**. The lower front part of the skull is formed by fourteen facial bones. Together with the cranium, the facial bones form spaces to hold the eyes, internal ear, nose, and mouth.

2. There are three **middle ear ossicles** in each ear, called the **malleus, incus,** and **stapes**, respectively, positioned between the eardrum and inner ear. They are among the smallest bones found in the human body. These bones transmit sounds from the air to the fluid-filled cochlea, and without them, individuals suffer from hearing loss.

3. The **hyoid bone** is a horseshoe-shaped bone located in the anterior midline of the neck. It is held in place by muscles and is only distantly articulated to other bones. It aids in swallowing and movement of the tongue.

4. The **rib cage** includes the **sternum,** or breastbone, and twelve pairs of **ribs.** The ribs each have one flat end and one rounded end, similar to a crescent shape. The flat ends of the upper seven ribs come together at the sternum, while their rounded ends are attached at joints to the vertebrae. The eighth, ninth, and tenth pairs of ribs connect to the ribs above with noncostal cartilage. The last two sets of ribs are floating ribs and do not attach to any other structure. The rib cage protects the heart and lungs.

5. The adult **vertebral column** comprises twenty-four vertebrae, the sacrum, and the coccyx. The **sacrum** is formed from five fused vertebrae, and the **coccyx** is formed from three to five fused vertebrae, so the vertebral column is thought to have thirty-three bones total. The seven cervical vertebrae are the

uppermost vertebrae and connect the cranium. Below the cervical vertebrae are twelve thoracic vertebrae, followed by five lumbar vertebrae.

Appendicular Skeleton

The appendicular skeleton comprises 126 bones that support the body's appendages. It helps with movement of the body as well as with manipulation of external objects and interactions with the environment. It is divided into the following four parts:

1. The pectoral girdles include four bones, which are the right and left clavicle and two scapula bones. The scapulae help keep the shoulders in place.

2. The upper limbs comprise the arms and the hands. The arms each consist of three bones. The humerus is in the upper part of the arm, and the ulna and radius are below the elbow, making up the forearm. The arm bones provide attachment points for muscles that allow for movement of the arms and wrist. Each hand has twenty-seven bones.

3. The pelvis comprises two coxal bones that provide an attachment point for the lower limbs and the axial skeleton.

4. The lower limbs comprise the legs, ankles, and feet. The legs are each made up of four bones. The femur is located in the thigh. The patella covers the knee. The tibia and fibula are in the lower leg below the knee. These bones have muscles attached to them that allow for movement of the leg. The foot and ankle of each leg have twenty-six bones total.

Functions of the Skeletal System

One of the major functions of the skeletal system is to provide structural support for the entire body. It provides a framework for the soft tissues and organs to attach to. The skeletal system also provides a reserve of important nutrients, such as calcium and lipids. Normal concentrations of calcium and phosphate in body fluids are partly maintained by the calcium salts stored in bone. Lipids that are stored in yellow bone marrow can be used as a source of energy. Red bone marrow produces red blood cells, white blood cells, and platelets that circulate in the blood. Certain groups of bones form protective barriers around delicate organs. The ribs, for example, protect the heart and lungs, the skull encloses the brain, and the vertebrae cover the spinal cord.

Compact and Spongy Bone

There are two types of bone: compact and spongy. **Compact bone** is dense with a matrix filled with organic substances and inorganic salts. There are only tiny spaces left between these materials for the **osteocytes**, or bone cells, to fit into. **Spongy bone**, in contrast to compact bone, is lightweight and porous. It covers the outside of the bone and gives it a shiny, white appearance. It has a branching network of parallel lamellae called **trabeculae**. Although spongy bone forms an open framework around the compact bone, it is still quite strong. Different bones have different ratios of compact to spongy bone depending on their function. The outside of the bone is covered by a **periosteum**, which has four major functions. It isolates and protects bones from the surrounding tissue, provides a place for attachment of the circulatory and nervous system structures, participates in growth and repair of the bone, and attaches the bone to the deep fascia. An **endosteum** is found inside the bone; it covers the trabeculae of the spongy bone and lines the inner surfaces of the central canals.

Life and Physical Sciences

Basic Macromolecules in a Biological System

There are six major elements found in most biological molecules: carbon, hydrogen, oxygen, nitrogen, sulfur, and phosphorus. These elements link together to make up the basic macromolecules of the biological system, which are lipids, carbohydrates, nucleic acids, and proteins. Most of these molecules use carbon as their backbone because of its ability to bond four different atoms. Each type of macromolecule has a specific structure and important function for living organisms.

Lipids

Lipids are made up of hydrocarbon chains, which are large molecules with hydrogen atoms attached to a long carbon backbone. These biological molecules are characterized as hydrophobic because their structure does not allow them to form bonds with water. When mixed together, the water molecules bond to each other and exclude the lipids. There are three main types of lipids: triglycerides, phospholipids, and steroids.

Triglycerides are made up of one glycerol molecule attached to three fatty acid molecules. **Glycerols** are three-carbon atom chains with one hydroxyl group attached to each carbon atom. **Fatty acids** are hydrocarbon chains with a backbone of sixteen to eighteen carbon atoms and a double-bonded oxygen molecule. Triglycerides have three main functions for living organisms. They are a source of energy when carbohydrates are not available, they help with absorption of certain vitamins, and they help insulate the body and maintain normal core temperature.

Phospholipid molecules have two fatty acid molecules bonded to one glycerol molecule, with the glycerol molecules having a phosphate group attached to it. The phosphate group has an overall negative charge, which makes that end of the molecule **hydrophilic,** meaning that it can bond with water molecules. Since the fatty acid tails of phospholipids are hydrophobic, these molecules are left with the unique characteristic of having different affinities on each of their ends. When mixed with water, phospholipids create **bilayers,** which are double rows of molecules with the hydrophobic ends on the inside facing each other and the hydrophilic ends on the outside, shielding the hydrophobic ends from the water molecules. Cells are protected by phospholipid bilayer cell membranes. This allows them to mix with aqueous solutions while also protecting their inner contents.

Steroids have a more complex structure than the other types of lipids. They are made up of four fused carbon rings. Different types of steroids are defined by the different chemical groups that attach to the carbon rings. Steroids are often mixed into phospholipid bilayers to help maintain the structure of the cell membrane and aid in cell signaling from these positions. They are also essential for regulation of metabolism and immune responses, among other biological processes.

Carbohydrates

Carbohydrates are made up of sugar molecules. **Monomers** are small molecules, and **polymers** are larger molecules that consist of repeating monomers. The smallest sugar molecule, or monosaccharide, has the chemical formula of CH_2O. Monosaccharides can be made up of one of these small molecules or a multiple of this formula (such as $C_2H_4O_2$). **Polysaccharides** consist of repeating monosaccharides in lengths of a few hundred to a few thousand linked together. Monosaccharides are broken down by living organisms to extract energy from the sugar molecules for immediate consumption. Glucose is a common monosaccharide used by the body as a primary energy source and which can be metabolized immediately. The more complex structure of polysaccharides allows them to have a more long-term use. They can be stored and broken down later for energy. Glycogen is a molecule that consists of 1700 to 600,000 glucose units linked together. It is not soluble in water and can be stored for long periods of time. If necessary, the glycogen molecule can be broken up into single glucose molecules in order to provide energy for the body. Polysaccharides also form structurally strong materials, such as chitin, which makes up the exoskeleton of many insects, and cellulose, which is the material that surrounds plant cells.

Nucleic Acids

Nucleotides are made up of a five-carbon sugar molecule with a nitrogen-containing base and one or more phosphate groups attached to it. **Nucleic acids** are polymers of nucleotides, or polynucleotides. There are two main types of nucleic acids: deoxyribonucleic acid (DNA) and ribonucleic acid (RNA). **DNA** is a double strand of nucleotides that are linked together and folded into a helical structure. Each strand is made up of four nucleotides, or bases: adenine, thymine, cytosine, and guanine. The adenine bases only pair with thymine on the opposite strand, and the cytosine bases only pair with guanine on the opposite strand. It is the links between these base pairs that create the helical structure of double-stranded DNA. DNA is in charge of long-term storage of genetic information that can be passed on to subsequent generations. It also contains instructions for constructing other components of the cell. **RNA,** on the other hand, is a single-stranded structure of nucleotides that is responsible for directing the construction of proteins within the cell. RNA is made up of three of the same nucleotides as DNA, but instead of thymine, adenine pairs with the base uracil.

Proteins

Proteins are made from a set of twenty amino acids that are linked together linearly, without branching. The amino acids have peptide bonds between them and form polypeptides. These polypeptide molecules coil up, either individually or as multiple molecules linked together, and form larger biological molecules, which are called proteins. Proteins have four distinct layers of structure. The primary structure consists of the sequence of amino acids. The secondary structure consists of the folds and coils formed by the hydrogen bonding that occurs between the atoms of the polypeptide backbone. The tertiary structure consists of the shape of the molecule, which comes from the interactions of the side chains that are linked to the polypeptide backbone. Lastly, the quaternary structure consists of the overall shape that the protein takes on when it is made up of two or more polypeptide chains. Proteins have many vital roles in living organisms. They help maintain and repair body tissue, provide a source of energy, form antibodies to aid the immune system, and are a large component in transporting molecules within the body, among many other functions.

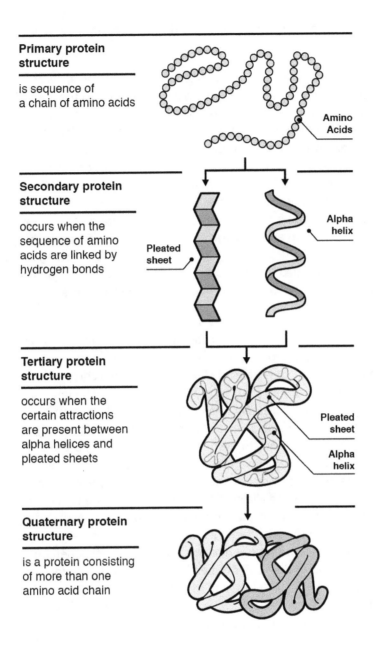

Primary protein structure

is sequence of a chain of amino acids

Amino Acids

Secondary protein structure

occurs when the sequence of amino acids are linked by hydrogen bonds

Pleated sheet

Alpha helix

Tertiary protein structure

occurs when the certain attractions are present between alpha helices and pleated sheets

Pleated sheet

Alpha helix

Quaternary protein structure

is a protein consisting of more than one amino acid chain

Comparing and Contrasting Chromosomes, Genes, and DNA

Chromosomes

A **chromosome** is a molecule of DNA that contains the genetic material of an organism, located in the nucleus of the cell. It is a threadlike structure made up of genes that is coiled tightly around proteins called **histones.** The histones support the more fragile form of the chromosome. Chromosomes are too small to even be seen under a microscope when a cell is not dividing. However, when a cell is undergoing division, the DNA making up the chromosomes becomes much more tightly packed and microscopically visible. During cell division, each chromosome makes an exact copy of itself that it is attached to at a constriction point called the **centromere.** The double chromosome structure, called **sister chromatids**, has an X shape, with one set of the chromosome's arms being longer than the other. In other words, the centromere is located closer to one end of the chromosome than the other. The shorter part of the chromosome sticking out from the centromere is called the **p-arm,** and the longer arm is called the **q-arm.**

For genetic information to be conserved from one generation to the next, chromosomes must be replicated and divided within the parent cell before being passed on to the daughter cell. Humans have twenty-three pairs of chromosomes. Twenty-two pairs are **autosomes,** or body chromosomes that contain most of the genetic hereditary information, and one pair is an **allosome,** or sex chromosome. Some genetic traits are sex-linked, so those genes are located on the allosome. Chromosomes are divided in humans during the process of meiosis. **Meiosis** is a special type of cell division in which a parent cell produces four daughter cells, each with half the number of chromosomes as the parent cell. As a precursor to meiosis, each chromosome replicates itself to form a sister chromatid. When a sperm cell meets an egg cell, each brings with it twenty-three sister chromatids. When meiosis starts, the homologous chromosomes pair up and undergo a crossing-over event where they can switch gene alleles. The remixed sister chromatids move toward the center of the cell along spindles and then are pulled to opposite poles and divided into two cells. These two cells divide again, breaking up the sister chromatids, and leaving each of the four cells with one set of chromosomes.

Genes

Genes are made up of DNA and are the basic functional unit of heredity. They can be as short as a few hundred DNA base pairs in length to over 2 million DNA base pairs long. Humans have between 20,000 and 25,000 genes on their twenty-three pairs of chromosomes. Each chromosome contains two **alleles,** or variations, of each gene—one inherited from each parent. Genes contain information about a specific trait that was inherited from one of the individual's parents. They provide instructions for making proteins to express that specific trait. Generally, one allele of a gene has a more dominant **phenotype,** or physical characteristic, than the other. This means that when both variations are present on a gene, the dominant variation or phenotype would always be expressed over the recessive phenotype. Since the dominant phenotype is always expressed when present, the recessive phenotype is only expressed when the gene only contains two recessive phenotype alleles. Although this is the case for almost all genes, some gene alleles have either codominance or incomplete dominance expression. With codominance, if both alleles are present, they are equally expressed in the phenotype. For example, certain cows can have red hair with two red hair alleles and white hair with two white hair alleles. However, when one of each allele is present, these cows have a mix of red and white hair on their bodies, not pink hair. Incomplete dominance occurs when two different alleles on a gene produce a third phenotype. For example, in certain types of flowers, two red alleles produce red flowers, and two white alleles produce white flowers. One of each allele produces pink flowers, a completely different color of flower.

Gene Mutations

Sometimes when genes are replicated, a permanent alteration in the DNA sequence occurs, and a gene mutation is formed. Mutations can be small and affect a single DNA base pair or be large and affect multiple genes in a chromosome. They can either be **hereditary,** which means they were present in the parent cell as well, or **acquired,** which means the mutation occurred at some point during cell replication within that individual's lifetime. Acquired mutations do not get passed on to subsequent generations. Most mutations are rare and occur in very small portions of the population. When the genetic alteration occurs in more than 1 percent of the population, it is called a **polymorphism.** Polymorphisms cause many of the variations seen in normal populations, such as hair and eye color, and do not affect a person's health. However, some polymorphisms put an individual at greater risk of developing some diseases.

DNA

DNA is the material that carries all of the hereditary information about an individual. It is present in every cell of the human body. DNA is a double-stranded molecule that coils up into a helical structure. Each strand is made from a sequence of four chemical bases, which are adenine, guanine, cytosine, and thymine. Each base pairs with only one of the four other bases when it is linked to the second strand—adenine with thymine and guanine with cytosine. The order of the base pairs and length of the strand determine what type of information is being coded. It varies for each gene that it makes up.

DNA Replication

An important characteristic of DNA is its ability to replicate itself. Each strand of the double-stranded DNA structure serves as a template for creating an exact replica of the DNA molecule. When cells divide, they require an exact copy of the DNA for the new cell. During DNA replication, the helical molecule is untwisted, and the strands are separated at one end. Specific replication proteins attach to each separated strand and begin forming new strands with matching base pairs for each of the strands. While some of the DNA molecule is untwisted, the remainder becomes increasingly twisted in response. Topoisomerase enzymes help relieve the strain of the excess twisting by breaking, untwisting, and rejoining the DNA strands. Once the replication proteins have copied the strands from one end to the other, two new DNA molecules are formed. Each DNA molecule is made from one original base pair strand and one newly synthesized base pair strand joined together.

Mendel's Laws of Heredity

Gregor Mendel was a monk who came up with one of the first models of inheritance in the 1860s. He is often referred to as the father of genetics. At the time, his theories were largely criticized because biologists did not believe that these ideas could be generally applicable and could also not apply to different species. They were later rediscovered in the early 1900s and given more credence by a group of European scientists. Mendel's original ideas have since been combined with other theories of inheritance to develop the ideas that are studied today.

Between 1856 and 1863, Gregor Mendel experimented with about five thousand pea plants that had different color flowers in his garden to test his theories of inheritance. He crossed purebred white flower and purple flower pea plants and found that the results were not a blend of the two flowers; they were instead all purple flowers. When he then fertilized this second generation of purple flowers with itself, both white flowers and purple flowers were produced, in a ratio of one to three. Although he used different terms at the time, he proposed that the color trait for the flowers was regulated by a gene, which he called a **factor,** and that there were two alleles, which he called **forms,** for each gene. For each gene, one allele was inherited from each parent. The results of these experiments allowed him to come up with his **Principles of Heredity**.

There are two main laws that Mendel developed after seeing the results of his experiments. The first law is the **Law of Segregation**, which states that each trait has two versions that can be inherited. In the parent cells, the allele pairs of each gene separate, or segregate, randomly during gamete production. Each gamete then carries only one allele with it for reproduction. During the process of reproduction, the gamete from each parent contributes its single allele to the daughter cell. The second law is the **Law of Independent Assortment,** which states that the alleles for different traits are not linked to one another and are inherited independently. It emphasizes that if a daughter cell selects allele A for gene 1, it does not also automatically select allele A for gene 2. The allele for gene 2 is selected in a separate, random manner.

Mendel theorized one more law, called the **Law of Dominance**, which has to do with the expression of a genotype but not with the inheritance of a trait. When he crossed the purple flower and white flower pea plants, he realized that the purple flowers were expressed at a greater ratio than the white flower pea plants. He hypothesized that certain gene alleles had a stronger outcome on the phenotype that was expressed. If a gene had two of the same allele, the phenotype associated with that allele was expressed. If a gene had two different alleles, the phenotype was determined by the dominant allele, and the other allele, the recessive allele, had no effect on the phenotype.

Basic Atomic Structure

Atoms are the smallest units of all matter and make up all chemical elements. They each have three parts: protons, neutrons, and electrons.

Measurable Properties of Atoms
Although atoms are very small in size, they have many properties that can be quantitatively measured. The **atomic mass** of an atom is equal to the sum of the protons and neutrons in the atom. The **ionization energy** of an atom is the amount of energy that is needed to remove one electron from an individual atom. The greater the ionization energy, the harder it is to remove the electron, meaning the greater the bond between the electron and that atom's nucleus. Ionization energies are always positive because atoms require extra energy to let go of an atom. On the other hand, **electron affinity** is the change in energy that occurs when an electron is added to an individual atom. Electron affinity is always negative because atoms release energy when an electron is added. The **effective nuclear charge** of an atom is noted as Z_{eff} and accounts for the attraction of electrons to the nucleus of an atom as well as the repulsion of electrons to other neighboring electrons in the same atom. The **covalent radius** of an atom is the radius of an atom when it is bonded to another atom. It is equal to one-half the distance between the two atomic nuclei. The **van der Waal's radius** is the radius of an atom when it is only colliding with another atom in solution or as a gas and is not bonding to the other atom.

The Periodic Table and Periodicity
Periodic Table
The **periodic table** is a chart that describes all the known elements. Currently, there are 118 elements listed on the periodic table. Each element has its own cell on the table. Within the cell, the element's abbreviation is written in the center, with its full name written directly below. The atomic number is recorded in the top left corner, and the atomic mass is recorded at the bottom center of the cell in atomic mass units, or **amus.** The first ninety-four elements are naturally occurring, whereas the last twenty-four can only be made in laboratory environments.

The rows of the table are called **periods,** and the columns are called **groups.** Elements with similar properties are grouped together. The periodic table can be divided and described in many ways according to similarities of the grouped elements. When it is divided into blocks, each block is named in accordance with the subshell in which the final electron sits. The blocks are named alkali metals, alkaline earth metals, transition metals, basic metals, semimetals, nonmetals, halogens, noble gases, lanthanides, and actinides. If the periodic table is divided according to shared physical and chemical properties, the elements are often classified as metals, metalloids, and nonmetals.

Periodicity
Periodicity refers to the trends that are seen in the periodic table among the elements. It is a fundamental aspect of how the elements are arranged within the table. These trends allow scientists to learn the properties of families of elements together instead of learning about each element only individually. They also elucidate the relationships among the elements. There are many important

characteristics that can be seen by examining the periodicity of the table, such as ionization energy, electron affinity, length of atomic radius, and metallic characteristics. Moving from left to right and from bottom to top on the periodic table, elements have increasing ionization energy and electron affinity. Moving in the opposite directions, from top to bottom and from right to left, the elements have increasing length of atomic radii. Moving from the bottom left corner to the top right corner, the elements have increasing nonmetallic properties, and moving in the opposite direction from the top right corner to the bottom left corner, the elements have increasing metallic properties.

Protons
Protons are found in the nucleus of an atom and have a positive electric charge. At least one proton is found in the nucleus of all atoms. Protons have a mass of about one atomic mass unit. The number of protons in an element is referred to as the element's atomic number. Each element has a unique number of protons and therefore its own unique atomic number. Hydrogen ions are unique in that they only contain one proton and do not contain any electrons. Since they are free protons, they have a very short lifespan and immediately become attracted to any free electrons in the environment. In a solution with water, they bind to a water molecule, H2O, and turn it into H3O+.

Neutrons
Neutrons are also found in the nucleus of atoms. These subatomic particles have a neutral charge, meaning that they do not have a positive or negative electric charge. Their mass is slightly larger than that of a proton. Together with protons, they are referred to as the nucleons of an atom. Interestingly, although neutrons are not affected by electric fields because of their neutral charge, they are affected by magnetic fields and are said to have magnetic moments.

Electrons
Electrons have a negative charge and are the smallest of the subatomic particles. They are located outside the nucleus in orbitals, which are shells that surround the nucleus. If an atom has an overall neutral charge, it has an equal number of electrons and protons. If it has more protons than electrons or vice versa, it becomes an **ion.** When there are more protons than electrons, the atom is a positively charged ion, or **cation.** When there are more electrons than protons, the atom is a negatively charged ion, or **anion.**

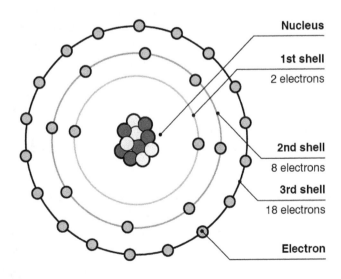

The location of electrons within an atom is more complicated than the locations of protons and neutrons. Within the orbitals, electrons are always moving. They can spin very fast and move upward, downward, and sideways. There are many different levels of orbitals around the atomic nucleus, and each orbital has a different capacity for electrons. The electrons in the orbitals closest to the nucleus are more tightly bound to the nucleus of the atom. There are three main characteristics that describe each orbital. The first is the **principle quantum number**, which describes the size of the orbital. The second is the **angular momentum quantum number**, which describes the shape of the orbital. The third is the **magnetic quantum number**, which describes the orientation of the orbital in space.

Chemical Bonds Between Atoms

Chemical bonds are formed from attractions between atoms that then create chemical compounds or molecules. The bonds can be strong or weak depending on how the bond is formed. A stable compound formed with the total energy of the molecular unit is lower than that of the atoms separately. There are many different types of chemical bonds that can form between atoms, including covalent bonds, ionic bonds, metallic bonds, and hydrogen bonds.

Covalent Bonds
An important characteristic of electrons is their ability to form covalent bonds with other atoms to form molecules. A covalent bond is a chemical bond that forms when two atoms share the same pair or pairs of electrons. There is a stable balance of attraction and repulsion between the two atoms. When these bonds are formed, energy is released because the electrons become more spatially distributed instead of being pulled toward the individual atom's nucleus. There are several different types of covalent bonds. **Sigma bonds** are the strongest type of covalent bond and involve the head-on overlapping of electron orbitals from two different atoms. **Pi bonds** are a little weaker and involve the lateral overlapping of certain orbitals. While single bonds between atoms, such as between carbon and hydrogen, are generally sigma bonds, double bonds, such as when carbon is double-bonded to an oxygen atom, are usually one sigma bond and one pi bond.

Covalent bonds can also be classified as nonpolar or polar. **Nonpolar covalent bonds** are formed when two atoms share their electrons equally, creating a very small difference of electronegativity between the atoms. Compounds that are formed with nonpolar covalent bonds do not mix well with water and other polar solvents and are much more soluble in nonpolar solvents. **Polar covalent bonds** are formed when electrons are not evenly shared between the atoms. Therefore, the electrons are pulled closer to one atom than the other, giving the molecule ionic properties and an imbalance of charge. The electronegative difference between the atoms is greater when polar bonds are formed compared to nonpolar bonds.

Coordinate covalent bonds, or **dipolar bonds**, are formed when the two shared electrons of the molecule come from the same atom. The electrons from one atom are shared with an empty orbital on the other atom, making one atom the electron pair donor and the other atom the electron pair acceptor. The electrons are shared approximately equally when these bonds are created.

Ionic Bonds
When ionic bonds are formed, instead of sharing a pair of electrons, the electrons are transferred from one atom to another, creating two ions. One of the ions is left with a positive charge, and the other one is left with a negative charge. This results in a large difference in electronegativity between the ions. The ionic bonds result from the attraction between the oppositely charged ions. However, the same two ions are not always paired with each other. Each ion is surrounded by ions with the opposite charge but are constantly moving around. Ionic bonds commonly form in metal salts. Metals have few electrons in their outermost orbitals, and by losing those electrons, they become more stable. By taking these electrons

away from the metallic atoms, nonmetals can fill their valence shells and also become more stable. For example, when sodium atoms and chloride atoms combine to form sodium chloride, the sodium atom loses an electron and becomes positively charged with a closed shell of electrons, and the chloride atom gains an electron, leaving it with a full shell of electrons.

Metallic Bonds

Metallic bonds occur when the electrons in the outer shell of an atom become delocalized and free-moving. They become shared by many atoms as they move in all directions around the positively charged metal ions. The free-floating electrons create an environment that allows for easy conduction of heat and electricity between the atoms. They also contribute to the **luster,** or surface reflectivity, that is often characteristic of metals, as well as the high tensile strength of metallic material. Metallic bonds are often seen as a sea of electrons with positive ions floating between them.

Hydrogen Bonds

Hydrogen bonds are different from the previously mentioned bonds because they are formed between a hydrogen atom that is present in one molecule and another atom that is already part of a molecular complex. These types of bonds are intermolecular instead of intramolecular. The hydrogen atom is attracted to an atom that has a high electronegativity in the other molecule. The large difference in electronegativity between the molecules creates a strong electrostatic attraction between the molecules. If a hydrogen atom forms a polar covalent bond with another atom, such as an oxygen atom, the hydrogen end of the molecule remains slightly positively charged, and the oxygen end of the molecule remains slightly negatively charged. The hydrogen of this molecule would then be attracted to other atoms with a slightly negative charge in nearby molecules. Hydrogen bonding is also important in the formation of the DNA double helix molecule. The nitrogenous bases on each strand are situated so they can form hydrogen bonds with the bases that are directly opposite them on the other strand.

Characteristic Properties of Substances

Properties of Water

Water is a polar compound formed from one oxygen atom bonded to two hydrogen atoms. It has many unique properties, such as its ability to exist as a solid, liquid, and gas on Earth's surface. It is the only common substance that can exist in all three forms in this environment. Water is also self-ionizing, breaking itself up into $H+$ and $OH-$ ions, which also makes it both an acid and a base.

The polarity of water and its attraction to other polar molecules is an important characteristic. **Cohesion** is the attraction of water molecules to each other. The slight negative charge of the oxygen atom in one molecule attracts the slightly positively charged hydrogen atoms of other water molecules. This attraction allows water to have surface tension. Insects, such as water striders, can actually walk across the surface of a pool of water. **Adhesion** is the attraction of water molecules to other molecules with which it can form hydrogen bonds. This attraction creates capillary action. **Capillary action** is the ability of water to "climb" up the side of a tube as it is attracted to the material of the tube. Its polarity also helps it break up ions in salts and bond to other polar substances, such as acids and alcohols. It is used to dissolve many substances and is often described as a **universal solvent** because of its polar attraction to other atoms and ions.

While most compounds become denser when they become solid, ice, the solid form of water, is actually less dense than the liquid form of water. The hydrogen bonds that form between the water molecules become ice crystals and more stable. The bonds remain spaced apart as the liquid freezes, creating a low density in the solid structure. Ice, therefore, floats to the top of a glass of liquid water.

Water is also a great moderator of temperature because of its high specific heat and high heat of vaporization. **Specific heat** is the amount of energy that is needed to change the temperature of one gram of a substance 1°C. When a substance has a high specific heat, it requires a lot of energy to change the temperature. Since water molecules form a lot of hydrogen bonds, it takes a lot of energy to break up the bonds. Since there are a lot of hydrogen bonds to absorb and release heat as they break and form, respectively, temperature changes are minimized. Similarly, **heat of vaporization** is the amount of energy needed to change 1 gram of liquid into gas. It takes a lot of energy to break the hydrogen bonds between liquid water molecules and turn them into water vapor.

Characteristic Properties of Molecules
There are two basic types of properties that can help characterize substances: physical and chemical. **Physical properties** can be detected without changing the substance's identity or composition. If a substance is subject to a physical change, its appearance changes, but its composition does not change at all. Common physical properties include color, odor, density, and hardness. Physical properties can also be classified as extensive or intensive. Extensive physical properties depend on the amount of substance that is present. These include characteristics such as mass and volume. Intensive properties do not depend on how much of the substance is present and remain the same regardless of quantity. These include characteristics such as density and color.

Chemical properties are characteristics of a substance that describe how it can be changed into a different chemical substance. A substance's composition is changed when it undergoes a chemical change. Chemical properties are measured and observed only as the substance is undergoing a change to become a different substance. Some examples of chemical properties are flammability, reactivity, toxicity, and ability to oxidize. These properties are detected by making changes to the substance's external environment and seeing how it reacts to the changes. An iron shovel that is left outside can become rusty. Rusting occurs when iron changes to iron oxide. While iron is very hard and a shiny silver color, iron oxide is flaky and a reddish-brown color. **Reactivity** is the ability of a substance to combine chemically with another substance. While some substances are very reactive, others are not reactive at all. For example, potassium is very reactive with water, and even a small amount causes an explosive reaction. Helium, on the other hand, does not react with any other substance.

It is often important to quantify the properties that are observed in a substance. Quantitative measurements are associated with a number, and it is imperative to include a unit of measure with each of those measurements. Without the unit of measure, the number may be meaningless. If the weight of a substance is noted as 100 without a unit of measure, it is unknown whether the substance is equivalent to 100 of something very light, such as milligram measurements, or 100 of something very heavy, such as kilogram measurements. There are many other quantitative measurements of matter that can be taken, including length, time, and temperature, among many others. Contrastingly, there are many properties that are not associated with a number; these properties can be measured qualitatively. The measurements of qualitative properties use a person's senses to observe and describe the characteristics. Since the descriptions are developed by individual persons, they can be very subjective. These properties can include odor, color, and texture, among many others. They can also include comparisons between two substances without using a number; for example, one substance may have a stronger odor or be lighter in color than another substance.

Changes in States of Matter

The universe is composed completely of matter. **Matter** is any material or object that takes up space and has a mass. Although there is an endless variety of items found in the universe, there are only about one hundred elements, or individual substances, that make up all matter. These elements are different types of atoms and are the smallest units that anything can be broken down into. Different elements can link together to form compounds, or molecules. Hydrogen and oxygen are two examples of elements, and when they bond together, they form water molecules. Matter can be found in three different states: gas, liquid, or solid.

Gases

Gases have three main distinct properties. The first is that they are easy to compress. When a gas is compressed, the space between the molecules decreases, and the frequency of collisions between them increases. The second property is that they do not have a fixed volume or shape. They expand to fill large containers or compress down to fit into smaller containers. When they are in large containers, the gas molecules can float around at high speeds and collide with each other, which allows them to fill the entire container uniformly. Therefore, the volume of a gas is generally equal to the volume of its container. The third distinct property of a gas is that it occupies more space than the liquid or solid from which it was formed. One gram of solid CO_2, also known as dry ice, has a volume of 0.641 milliliters. The same amount of CO_2 in a gaseous state has a volume of 556 milliliters. Steam engines use water in this capacity to do work. When water boils inside the steam engine, it becomes steam, or water vapor. As the steam increases in volume and escapes its container, it is used to make the engine run.

Liquids

A liquid is an intermediate state between gases and solids. It has an exact volume due to the attraction of its molecules to each other and molds to the shape of the part of the container that it is in. Although liquid molecules are closer together than gas molecules, they still move quickly within the container they are in. Liquids cannot be compressed, but their molecules slide over each other easily when poured out of a container. The attraction between liquid molecules, known as **cohesion,** also causes liquids to have surface tension. They stick together and form a thin skin of particles with an extra strong bond between them. As long as these bonds remain undisturbed, the surface becomes quite strong and can even support the weight of an insect such as a water skipper. Another property of liquids is **adhesion,** which is when different types of particles are attracted to each other. When liquids are in a container, they are drawn up above the surface level of the liquid around the edges. The liquid molecules that are in contact with the container are pulled up by their extra attraction to the particles of the container.

Solids

Unlike gases and liquids, solids have a definitive shape. They are similar to liquids in that they also have a definitive volume and cannot be compressed. The molecules are packed together tightly, which does not allow for movement within the substance. There are two types of solids: crystalline and amorphous. **Crystalline solids** have atoms or molecules arranged in a specific order or symmetrical pattern throughout the entire solid. This symmetry makes all of the bonds within the crystal of equal strength, and when they are broken apart, the pieces have straight edges. Minerals are all crystalline solids. **Amorphous solids**, on the other hand, do not have repeating structures or symmetry. Their components are heterogeneous, so they often melt gradually over a range of temperatures. They do not break evenly and often have curved edges. Examples of amorphous solids are glass, rubber, and most plastics.

Matter can change between a gas, liquid, and solid. When these changes occur, the change is physical and does not affect the chemical properties or makeup of the substance. Environmental changes, such as temperature or pressure changes, can cause one state of matter to convert to another state of matter. For example, in very hot temperatures, solids can melt and become a liquid, such as when ice melts into liquid water, or sublimate and become a gas, such as when dry ice becomes gaseous carbon dioxide. Liquids can evaporate and become a gas, such as when liquid water turns into water vapor. In very cold temperatures, gases can depose and become a solid, such as when water vapor becomes icy frost on a windshield, or condense and become a liquid, such as when water vapor becomes dew on grass. Liquids can freeze and become a solid, such as when liquid water freezes and becomes ice.

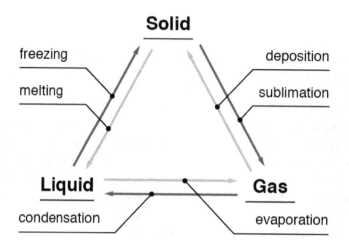

Chemical Reactions

A chemical reaction is a process that involves a change in the molecular arrangement of a substance. Generally, one set of chemical substances, called the reactants, is rearranged into a different set of chemical substances, called the products, by the breaking and re-forming of bonds between atoms. In a chemical reaction, it is important to realize that no new atoms or molecules are introduced. The products are formed solely from the atoms and molecules that are present in the reactants. These can involve a change in state of matter as well. Making glass, burning fuel, and brewing beer are all examples of chemical reactions.

Types of Chemical Reactions
Generally, chemical reactions are thought to involve changes in positions of electrons with the breaking and re-forming of chemical bonds, without changes to the nucleus of the atoms. The three main types of chemical reactions are combination, decomposition, and combustion.

Combination
In combination reactions, two or more reactants are combined to form one more complex, larger product. The bonds of the reactants are broken, the elements rearranged, and then new bonds are formed between all of the elements to form the product. It can be written as A + B → C, where A and B are the reactants and C is the product. An example of a combination reaction is the creation of iron(II) sulfide from iron and sulfur, which is written as $8Fe + S_8 \rightarrow 8FeS$.

Decomposition
Decomposition reactions are almost the opposite of combination reactions. They occur when one substance is broken down into two or more products. The bonds of the first substance are broken, the elements rearranged, and then the elements bonded together in new configurations to make two or more molecules. These reactions can be written as C → B + A, where C is the reactant and A and B are the products. An example of a decomposition reaction is the electrolysis of water to make oxygen and hydrogen gas, which is written as $2H_2O \rightarrow 2H_2 + O_2$.

Combustion

Combustion reactions are a specific type of chemical reaction that involves oxygen gas as a reactant. This mostly involves the burning of a substance. The combustion of hexane in air is one example of a combustion reaction. The hexane gas combines with oxygen in the air to form carbon dioxide and water. The reaction can be written as $2C_6H_{14} + 17O_2 \rightarrow 12CO_2 + 14H_2O$.

Balancing Chemical Reactions

The way the hexane combustion reaction is written above ($2C_6H_{14} + 17O_2 \rightarrow 12CO_2 + 14H_2O$) is an example of a chemical equation. Chemical equations describe how the molecules are changed when the chemical reaction occurs. The "+" sign on the left side of the equation indicates that those molecules are reacting with each other, and the arrow, "$\rightarrow$," in the middle of the equation indicates that the reactants are producing something else. The coefficient before a molecule indicates the quantity of that specific molecule that is present for the reaction. The subscript next to an element indicates the quantity of that element in each molecule. In order for the chemical equation to be balanced, the quantity of each element on both sides of the equation should be equal. For example, in the hexane equation above, there are twelve carbon elements, twenty-eight hydrogen elements, and thirty-four oxygen elements on each side of the equation. Even though they are part of different molecules on each side, the overall quantity is the same. The state of matter of the reactants and products can also be included in a chemical equation and would be written in parentheses next to each element as follows: gas (g), liquid (l), solid (s), and dissolved in water, or aqueous (aq).

Catalysts

The rate of a chemical reaction can be increased by adding a catalyst to the reaction. Catalysts are substances that lower the activation energy required to go from the reactants to the products of the reaction but are not consumed in the process. The **activation energy** of a reaction is the minimum amount of energy that is required to make the reaction move forward and change the reactants into the products. When catalysts are present, less energy is required to complete the reaction. For example, hydrogen peroxide will eventually decompose into two water molecules and one oxygen molecule. If potassium permanganate is added to the reaction, the decomposition happens at a much faster rate. Similarly, increasing the temperature or pressure in the environment of the reaction can increase the rate of the reaction. Higher temperatures increase the number of high-energy collisions that lead to the products. The same happens when increasing pressure for gaseous reactants, but not with solid or liquid reactants.

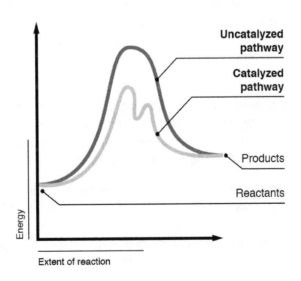

Enzymes

Enzymes are a type of biological catalyst that accelerate chemical reactions. They work like other catalysts by lowering the activation energy of the reaction to increase the reaction rate. They bind to substrates and change them into the products of the reaction without being consumed by the reaction. Enzymes differ from other catalysts by their increased specificity to their substrate. They can also be affected by other molecules. Enzyme inhibitors can decrease their activity, whereas enzyme activators increase their activity. Their activity also decreases dramatically when the environment is not in their optimal pH and temperature range.

An enzyme can encounter several different types of inhibitors. In biological systems, inhibitors are many times expressed as part of a feedback loop where the enzyme is producing too much of a substance too quickly and the reaction needs to be stopped. **Competitive inhibitors** and substrates cannot bind to the enzyme at the same time. These inhibitors often resemble the substrate of the enzyme. Noncompetitive inhibitors bind to the enzyme at a different location than the substrate. The substrate can still bind with the same affinity, but the efficiency of the enzyme is decreased. **Uncompetitive inhibitors** cannot bind to the enzyme alone and can only bind to the enzyme–substrate complex. Once an uncompetitive inhibitor binds to the complex, the complex becomes inactive. An **irreversible inhibitor** binds to the enzyme and permanently inactivates it. It usually does so by forming a covalent bond with the enzyme.

pH

In chemistry, **pH** stands for the potential of hydrogen. It is a numeric scale ranging from 0 to 14 that determines the acidity and basicity of an aqueous solution. Solutions with a pH of greater than 7 are considered basic, those with a pH of less than 7 are considered acidic, and solutions with a pH equal to 7 are considered neutral. Pure water is considered neutral with a pH equal to 7. It is important to remember that the pH of solutions can change at different temperatures. While the pH of pure water is 7 at 25°C, at 0°C it is 7.47, and at 100°C it is 6.14. pH is calculated as the negative of the base 10 logarithm of the activity of the hydrogen ions in the solution and can be written as $pH = -\log_{10}(a_H+) = \log_{10}(1/a_H+)$.

One of the simplest ways to measure the pH of a solution is by performing a litmus test. Litmus paper has a mixture of dyes on it that react with the solution and display whether the solution is acidic or basic depending on the resulting color. Red litmus paper turns blue when it reacts with a base. Blue litmus paper turns red when it reacts with an acid. Litmus tests are generally crude measurements of pH and not very precise. A more precise way to measure the pH of a solution is to use a pH meter. These specialized meters act like voltmeters and measure the electrical potential of a solution. Acids have a lot of positively charged hydrogen ions in solutions that have greater potential than bases to produce an electric current. The voltage measurement is then compared with a solution of known pH and voltage. The difference in voltage is translated into the difference in pH.

Acids and Bases

Acids and bases are two types of substances with differing properties. In general, when acids are dissolved in water, they can conduct electricity, have a sour taste, react with metals to free hydrogen ions, and react with bases to neutralize their properties. Bases, in general, when dissolved in water, conduct electricity, have a slippery feel, and react with acids to neutralize their properties.

The Brønsted-Lowry acid–base theory is a commonly accepted theory about how acid–base reactions work. **Acids** are defined as substances that dissociate in aqueous solutions and form hydrogen ions. **Bases** are defined as substances that dissociate in aqueous solutions and form hydroxide (OH^-) ions. The basic idea behind the theory is that when an acid and base react with each other, a proton is exchanged, and the acid forms its conjugate base, while the base forms its conjugate acid. The acid is the proton donor,

146

and the base is the proton acceptor. The reaction is written as HA + B ↔ A⁻ + HB⁺, where HA is the acid, B is the base, A⁻ is the conjugated base, and HB⁺ is the conjugated acid. Since the reverse of the reaction is also possible, the reactants and products are always in equilibrium. The equilibrium of acids and bases in a chemical reaction can be determined by finding the acid dissociation constant, K_a, and the base dissociation constant, K_b. These dissociation constants determine how strong the acid or base is in the aqueous solution. Strong acids and bases dissociate quickly to create the products of the reaction.

In other cases, acids and bases can react to form a neutral salt. This happens when the hydrogen ion from the acid combines with the hydroxide ion of the base to form water, and the remaining ions combine to form a neutral salt. For example, when hydrochloric acid and sodium hydroxide combine, they form salt and water, which can be written as $HCl + NaOH \rightarrow NaCl + H_2O$.

Scientific Reasoning

Identifying Basic Scientific Measurement Using Laboratory Tools

Measuring Force

A Newton meter or force meter is a standardized instrument for measuring the force exerted by different elements in the universe that cause movement when they act upon objects by pulling, pushing, rotating, deforming, or accelerating them, such as gravity, friction, or tension. Force is measured in units called Newtons (N), named after Sir Isaac Newton, who defined the laws of motion, including forces. One common example of a force meter is a bathroom scale. When someone steps on the scale, the force exerted on the platform is measured in the form of units of weight. Force meters contain springs, rubber bands, or other elastic materials that stretch in proportion to force applied. A Newton meter displays 50-Newton increments, with four 10-Newton marks in between. Thus if a Newton meter's needle rests on the third mark between 100 and 150, this indicates 130N.

Measuring Temperature

As those familiar with word roots can determine, thermometers measure heat or temperature (*thermo-* is from Greek for heat and *meter* from Greek for measure). Some thermometers measure outdoor or indoor air temperature, and others measure body temperature in humans or animals. Meat thermometers measure temperature in the center of cooked meat to ensure sufficient cooking to kill bacteria. Refrigerator and freezer thermometers measure internal temperatures to ensure sufficient coldness. Although digital thermometers eliminate the task of reading a thermometer scale by displaying a specific numerical reading, many thermometers still use visual scales. In these, increments are typically two-tenths of a degree. However, basal thermometers, which are more sensitive and accurate, and are frequently used to track female ovulation cycles for measuring and planning fertility, display increments of one-tenth of a degree. Whole degrees are marked by their numbers; tenths of degrees are the smallest marks in between.

Measuring Length

Rulers, yardsticks, tape measures, and other standardized instruments are for measuring short distances. Standard rulers and similar measures show distances in increments of feet, inches, and halves, quarters, eights, and sixteenths of an inch. Tape measures have markings indicating one yard or three feet, six feet, and other common multiple-feet measurements. Each inch on a ruler is marked by number from 1 to 12 (or 1 to 36 on a yardstick). Half-inches are the longest of the non-numbered line marks, then quarter-inches, then eighth-inches, then sixteenth-inches. Some American-made rulers also include metric measurements.

Using the Vernier Scale

French mathematician and inventor Pierre Vernier originated the Vernier measurement principle and corresponding scale in 1631. When measuring small increments using other instruments, it can be impossible to determine precisely small fractions within already small divisions. Vernier's invention solved this problem with simple elegance. For example, dividing millimeters in the metric system or 16ths of an inch in the English system into 10ths or smaller portions is impractical, inaccurate, and unreadable without using magnifiers. A metric Vernier caliper features a main scale and a Vernier scale, i.e. a parallel, sliding scale with ten or eleven marks, spaced equally within themselves but differently from the main scale spacing. English Vernier calipers often have $\frac{1}{16}$" main scale divisions and 8 divisions on the Vernier scale, so they can measure lengths as small as $\frac{1}{28}$". To read a Vernier caliper, close its jaws on the object being measured, note the main scale number, rounding down to the next smaller marking, and see which Vernier scale mark aligns with it to obtain the additional fraction.

Using a Micrometer Caliper

A micrometer caliper is similar to a Vernier caliper in that both have a main scale plus a movable scale for measuring fractions of small numbers. Like many medical instruments, micrometer calipers are typically metrical, measuring in millimeters. The main scale markings are in $\frac{1}{2}$ millimeters. A uniform, precise screw moves the micrometer caliper's jaw. It has a rotating thimble on its handle, marked in 50 equal divisions. Rotating the thimble once moves the screw $\frac{1}{2}$ millimeter along the main scale, enabling the user to read measurements as small as one-hundredth of a millimeter. Most micrometers display $\frac{1}{2}$ mm markings on the thimble on the opposite side from the main scale markings on the micrometer sleeve, making it easier to read. Users require some practice, e.g. rounding up $\frac{1}{2}$ mm if a reading is in the top half of a millimeter; only tightening the caliper jaws using the slip clutch to close them snugly without bending them; and making a zero correction using a special wrench so fully closing the jaws yields a zero reading if it did not already.

Critiquing a Scientific Explanation Using Logic and Evidence

According to the scientific method, one must either observe something as it is happening or as a constant state, or prove it through experimenting, to say it is a fact. Scientific experiments are found reliable when they can be replicated and produce comparable results regardless of who is conducting them or making the observations. However, historically many beliefs have been considered facts at the time, only to be disproven later when objective evidence became accessible. For instance, in ancient times many people believed the Earth was flat based on limited visual evidence. Ancient Greek philosophers Pythagoras in the 6th century BCE and Aristotle in the 4th century BCE believed the earth was spherical. This was eventually borne out by observational evidence. Aristotle estimated the Earth's circumference; Eratosthenes measured it c. 240 BCE; in the 2nd century CE, Ptolemy had mapped the globe and developed the latitude, longitude, and climes system.

While many phenomena have been established by science as facts, technically many others are actually theories, though many people mistakenly consider them facts. As one example, gravity per se is a fact; however, the scientific explanation of how gravity functions is a theory. Though a theory is not the same as a fact, this does not presume theories are merely speculative ideas. A scientific theory must be tested thoroughly and then applied to established facts, hypotheses, and observations. Moreover, for a theory to be accepted or even considered scientifically, it must relate and explain a broad scope of observations which would not be related without the theory. People sometimes state opinions as if they were facts to persuade others. For example, advertising might claim a product is the best without concrete supporting

148

evidence. To evaluate information, one must consider both its source and any supporting evidence to ascertain its veracity.

Relationships Among Events, Objects, and Procedures

When we determine relationships among events, objects, and procedures, we are better able to understand the world around us and make predictions based on that understanding. With regards to relationships among events and procedures, we will look at cause and effect. For relationships among objects, we will take a look at Newton's Laws.

Cause
The **cause** of a particular event is the thing that brings it about. A causal relationship may be partly or wholly responsible for its effect, but sometimes it's difficult to tell whether one event is the sole cause of another event. For example, lung cancer can be caused by smoking cigarettes. However, sometimes lung cancer develops even though someone does not smoke, and that tells us that there may be other factors involved in lung cancer besides smoking. It's also easy to make mistakes when considering causation. One common mistake is mistaking correlation for causation. For example, say that in the year 2008 a volcano erupted in California, and in that same year, the number of infant deaths increased by ten percent. If we automatically assume, without looking at the data, that the erupting volcano *caused* the infant deaths, then we are mistaking correlation for causation. The two events might have happened at the same time, but that does not necessarily mean that one event caused the other. Relationships between events are never absolute; there are a myriad of factors that can be traced back to their foundations, so we must be thorough with our evidence in proving causation.

Effect
An **effect** is the result of something that occurs. For example, the Nelsons have a family dog. Every time the dog hears thunder, the dog whines. In this scenario, the thunder is the cause, and the dog's whining is the effect. Sometimes a cause will produce multiple effects. Let's say we are doing an experiment to see what the effects of exercise are in a group of people who are not usually active. After about four weeks, the group experienced weight loss, rise in confidence, and higher energy. We start out with a cause: exercising more. From that cause, we have three known effects that occurred within the group: weight loss, rise in confidence, and higher energy. Cause and effect are important terms to understand when conducting scientific experiments.

Newton's Laws
Newton's laws of motion describe the relationship between an object and the forces acting upon that object, and its movement responding to those forces. Newton has three laws:

Law of Inertia: An object at rest stays at rest and an object in motion stays in motion unless otherwise acted upon by an outside force. For example, gravity is an outside force that will affect the speed and direction of a ball; when we throw a ball, the ball will eventually decrease in speed and fall to the ground because of the outside force of gravity. However, if the ball were kicked in space where there is no gravity, the ball would go the same speed and direction forever unless it hits another object in space or falls into another gravity field.

Newton's Second Law: This law states that the heavier an object, the more force has to be used to move it. This force has to do with acceleration. For example, if you use the same amount of force to push both a golf cart and an eighteen-wheeler, the golf cart will have more acceleration than the truck because the eighteen-wheeler weighs more than the golf cart.

Newton's Third Law: This law states that for every action, there is an opposite and equal reaction. For example, if you are jumping on a trampoline, you are experiencing Newton's third law of motion. When you jump down on the trampoline, the opposite reaction pushes you up into the air.

Design of a Scientific Investigation

Scientific investigation is seeking an answer to a specific question using the scientific method. The scientific method is a procedure that is based on an observation. For example, if someone observes something strange, and they want to understand the process, they might ask how that process works. If we were to use the scientific method to understand the process, we would formulate a hypothesis. A hypothesis explains what you expect to happen from the experiment. Then, an experiment is conducted, data from the experiment is analyzed, and a conclusion is reached. Below are steps of the scientific method in a practical situation:

- Observation: One day, a student observes that every time he eats a big lunch, he falls asleep in the next period.

- Experimental Question: The question the student asks is, what is the relationship between eating large meals and energy levels?

- Formulate a Hypothesis: The student hypothesizes that eating a big meal will lead to lower energy due to the body using its energy to digest the food.

- Conduct an Experiment (Materials and Procedure): The student has his whole class eat two meals for lunch for a week, then he measures their energy levels in the next period. The next week, the student has them eat a small lunch, and then measures their energy levels in the next period.

- Analyze Data: The data in the student's experiment showed that in the first week, sixty percent of the students felt sleepy in the next period class and that in the second week, only twenty percent of the students felt sleepy in the next period class.

- Conclusion: The student concluded that the data supported his hypothesis: student energy levels decrease after the consumption of a large meal.

An important component of scientific research after the experiment is conducted is called peer review. This is when the article written about the experiment is sent to other scientists to "review." The reviewers offer feedback so that the editors can decide whether or not to publish the findings in a scholarly or scientific journal.

Practice Questions

1. How many different types of cells are there in the human body?
    a. Two hundred
    b. One thousand
    c. Ten
    d. Twenty-five

    (answer marked: A)

2. What type of tissue provides a protective barrier for delicate organs?
    a. Epithelial
    b. Muscle
    c. Connective
    d. Neural

    (answer marked: C)

3. What part of the respiratory system is responsible for regulating the temperature and humidity of the air that comes into the body?
    a. Larynx
    b. Lungs
    c. Trachea
    d. Sinuses *(circled)*

4. True or False: Carbon dioxide-rich blood returns to the heart to get pumped through the systemic circuit.
    a. False *(circled)*
    b. True

5. Which organ is responsible for gas exchange between air and circulating blood?
    a. Nose
    b. Larynx
    c. Lungs *(circled)*
    d. Stomach

6. Which layer of the heart wall contains nerves?
    a. Epicardium
    b. Myocardium
    c. Endocardium *(circled)*
    d. Sternum

7. What is another name for the mitral valve?
    a. Bicuspid valve *(circled)*
    b. Pulmonary valve
    c. Aortic valve
    d. Tricuspid valve

8. Which component of blood helps to fight off diseases?
    a. Red blood cells
    b. White blood cells *(circled)*
    c. Plasma
    d. Platelets

9. Which system consists of a group of organs that work together to transform food and liquids into fuel for the body?
    a. Respiratory system
    b. Immune system
    c. Genitourinary system
    d. Gastrointestinal system

10. There are multiple steps that the gastrointestinal system performs. In which step do chemicals and enzymes break down complex food molecules into smaller molecules?
    a. Digestion
    b. Absorption
    c. Compaction
    d. Ingestion

11. Which accessory organ of the gastrointestinal system is responsible for storing and concentrating bile?
    a. Liver
    b. Pancreas
    c. Stomach
    d. Gallbladder

12. Which type of muscle helps pump blood through the veins and arteries?
    a. Skeletal
    b. Smooth
    c. Intestinal
    d. Cardiac

13. How do neuroglia support neurons?
    a. Provide nutrition to them
    b. Provide a framework around them and protect them from the surrounding environment
    c. Relay messages to them from the brain
    d. Connect them to other surrounding cells

14. Which nerve system allows the brain to regulate body functions such as heart rate and blood pressure?
    a. Central
    b. Somatic
    c. Autonomic
    d. Afferent

15. Which of the following organs is NOT considered an accessory organ of the male reproductive system?
    a. Testes
    b. Prostate
    c. Vas deferens
    d. Bulbourethral glands

16. How many gametes do the ovaries produce every month?
    a. One million
    b. One
    c. One-half billion
    d. Two

17. In what part of the female reproductive system do sperm fertilize an oocyte?
    a. Ovary
    b. Mammary gland
    c. Vagina
    d. Fallopian tubes

18. What is the largest organ in the human body?
    a. Brain
    b. Large intestine
    c. Skin
    d. Heart

19. Which is a function of the skin?
    a. Temperature regulation
    b. Breathing
    c. Ingestion
    d. All of the above

20. Which accessory organ of the integumentary system provides a hard layer of protection over the skin?
    a. Hair
    b. Nails
    c. Sweat glands
    d. Sebaceous glands

21. Which is a distinct characteristic of tissues and glands that are a part of the endocrine system?
    a. Lack a blood supply
    b. Act quickly in response to stimuli
    c. Secrete bile
    d. Ductless

22. Which endocrine gland is found at the bottom of the hypothalamus?
    a. Pituitary
    b. Thymus
    c. Thyroid
    d. Pancreas

23. Which endocrine gland regulates the blood sugar levels of the body?
    a. Pineal
    b. Parathyroid
    c. Pancreas
    d. Adrenal

24. Which organ is responsible for filtering waste products out of the bloodstream?
    a. Kidneys
    b. Urinary bladder
    c. Pancreas
    d. Urethra

25. True or false: The genital system and urinary system have a shared pathway in males.
    a. True
    b. False

26. What happens to the urinary bladder as urine enters and is stored until the bladder is emptied?
    a. Blood flow to the organ increases.
    b. It secretes waste into the urine.
    c. Its walls stretch and become thinner.
    d. Its internal pressure increases.

27. Which immune system works in a nonspecific way and does not remember pathogens that it previously fought against?
    a. Innate
    b. Adaptive
    c. Hormonal
    d. B cell

28. How does the adaptive immune system work to fight against previously encountered pathogens?
    a. It sends out all antibodies to inactivate the pathogen.
    b. It sends out target-specific antibodies to inactivate the pathogen.
    c. It uses a mechanical barrier, such as the skin, to protect against pathogens.
    d. It uses a chemical barrier, such as gastric acid, to protect against pathogens.

29. What type of disorder can develop if the immune system is not functioning properly?
    a. Adaptive
    b. Innate
    c. Lymphocytic
    d. Autoimmune

30. How many bones are in the adult human skeletal system?
    a. 206
    b. Three hundred
    c. Twenty-seven
    d. Twenty-six

31. Which is a distinct characteristic of spongy bone?
    a. Dense
    b. Filled with organic and inorganic salts
    c. Found inside compact bone
    d. Lightweight

32. Which is NOT an example of a group of bones that forms a protective barrier around delicate organs?
    a. Foot bones
    b. Skull
    c. Ribs
    d. Vertebrae

33. Which molecule is the simplest form of sugar?
    a. Monosaccharide
    b. Fatty acid
    c. Polysaccharide
    d. Amino acid

34. Which type of macromolecule contains genetic information that can be passed to subsequent generations?
    a. Carbohydrates
    b. Lipids
    c. Proteins
    d. Nucleic acids

35. What is the primary unit of inheritance between generations of an organism?
    a. Chromosome
    b. Gene
    c. Gamete
    d. Atom

36. Which one of Mendel's laws theorizes that the alleles for different traits are NOT linked and can be inherited independently of one another?
    a. The Law of Dominance
    b. The Law of Segregation
    c. The Law of Independent Assortment
    d. None of the above

37. In which situation is an atom considered neutral?
    a. The number of protons and neutrons are equal.
    b. The number of neutrons and electrons are equal.
    c. The number of protons and electrons are equal.
    d. There are more electrons than protons.

38. Which is an example of a physical property of substances?
    a. Odor
    b. Reactivity
    c. Flammability
    d. Toxicity

39. Which type of matter has molecules that cannot move within its substance and breaks evenly across a plane caused by the symmetry of its molecular arrangement?
    a. Gas
    b. Crystalline solid
    c. Liquid
    d. Amorphous solid

40. What type of reactions involve the breaking and re-forming of bonds between atoms?
    a. Chemical
    b. Physical
    c. Isotonic
    d. Electron

41. What is the instrument used for measuring the force exerted by different elements in the universe that cause movement when they act upon objects by pulling, pushing, rotating, deforming, or accelerating them?
    a. Isaac force
    b. Newton meter
    c. Micrometer Caliper
    d. Vernier Scale

42. Which of the following describes an invention used to measure small fractions within already small divisions?
    a. A tape measure
    b. A ruler
    c. A yardstick
    d. Vernier Scale

43. When are scientific experiments found reliable?
    a. When all the materials needed for the experiment are used
    b. When the scientists conducting them are credible
    c. When they prove the hypothesis to be true
    d. When they can be replicated

44. Which of the following scenarios describes mistaking correlation for causation?
    a. In the same year, the drinking water was contaminated by a nearby chicken farm and stomach cancer in the area increased 3 percent. The contaminated water obviously caused stomach cancer to increase.
    b. Victoria notices that every time she turns on the stove burner underneath a pot with water in it, the water boils. Victoria realizes that putting heat under water causes it to boil.
    c. We saw that the thunderstorm that day caused all the neighborhoods in the East Village to flood. We could hardly get to the movie that night because of all the rain!
    d. Hector learned in school that when tectonic plates shift, it causes earthquakes to happen. There had been many earthquakes when Hector lived in California, and now he knew that the shifting of plates is what caused them.

45. Harley's sister, Camille, is pushing her on the swing. Camille notices that every time she pushes Camille forward, the swing propels back just as far. This is an example of which of the following of laws?
    a. Law of Inertia
    b. Newton's Second Law
    c. Newton's Third Law
    d. Law of Segregation

46. In the model of the scientific method, which of the following best explains the step of formulating a hypothesis?
    a. Forming a question that relates to the observation.
    b. Writing out an expectation of what's going to happen.
    c. Gathering the materials needed for the procedure.
    d. Summarizing the results of the experiment.

47. When would a peer review be conducted in an experiment?
    a. Before the experiment.
    b. During the experiment.
    c. After the experiment is over and before it is published.
    d. After the experiment is over and published.

Answer Explanations

1. A: There are only two hundred different types of cells in the human body. While there are trillions of cells that make up the human body, only two hundred different types make up that trillion, each with a specific function.

2. C: Connective tissue is located only on the inside of the body and fills internal spaces. This allows it to protect the organs within the body. Epithelial tissue is found on the outside of the body and as a lining of internal cavities and passageways. Muscle tissue allows for movement of the body. Neural tissue sends information from the brain to the rest of the body through electrical impulses.

3. D: After air enters the nose or mouth, it gets passed on to the sinuses. The sinuses regulate temperature and humidity before passing the air on to the rest of the body. Volume of air can change with varying temperatures and humidity levels, so it is important for the air to be a constant temperature and humidity before being processed by the lungs. The larynx is the voice box of the body, making Choice *A* incorrect. The lungs are responsible for oxygen and carbon dioxide exchange between the air that is breathed in and the blood that is circulating the body, making Choice *B* incorrect. The trachea takes the temperature- and humidity-regulated air from the sinuses to the lungs, making Choice *C* incorrect.

4. A: False. The blood needs to be oxygen-rich for the body to function properly. Oxygen-rich blood goes from the lungs to the heart and then is pumped through the systemic circuit to the rest of the body. Carbon dioxide-rich blood goes from the heart to the lungs, where the carbon dioxide is removed from the blood and breathed out of the body.

5. C: The main function of the lungs is to provide oxygen to the blood circulating in the body and to remove carbon dioxide from blood that has already circulated the body. The passageways within the lungs are responsible for this gas exchange between the air and the blood. The nose, Choice *A*, is the first place where air is breathed in. The larynx, Choice *B*, is the voice box of the body. The stomach, Choice *D*, is responsible for getting nutrients out of food and drink that are ingested, not from air.

6. B: The myocardium is the middle layer of the heart wall and contains connective tissue, blood vessels, and nerves. The epicardium, Choice *A*, is the outer layer of the heart wall and is solely made up of a serous membrane without any nerves or blood vessels. The endocardium, Choice *C*, is the inner layer of the heart wall and is made up of a simple squamous epithelium. The sternum, Choice *D*, is the chest bone and protects the heart.

7. A: The mitral valve is also known as the bicuspid valve because it has two leaflets. It is located on the left side of the heart between the atrium and the ventricle. The pulmonary valve, Choice *B*, is located between the right ventricle and the pulmonary artery and has three cusps. The aortic valve, Choice *C*, is located between the left ventricle and the aorta and also has three cusps. The tricuspid valve, Choice *D*, has three leaflets and is located on the right side of the heart between the atrium and the ventricle.

8. B: White blood cells are part of the immune system and help fight off diseases. Red blood cells contain hemoglobin, which carries oxygen through the blood. Plasma is the liquid matrix of the blood. Platelets help with the clotting of the blood.

9. D: The gastrointestinal system comprises the stomach and intestines, which help process food and liquid so that the body can absorb nutrients for fuel. The respiratory system is involved with the exchange of oxygen and carbon dioxide between the air and blood. The immune system helps the body fight against pathogens and diseases. The genitourinary system helps the body to excrete waste.

10. A: During digestion, complex food molecules are broken down into smaller molecules so that nutrients can be isolated and absorbed by the body. Absorption, Choice *B*, is when vitamins, electrolytes, organic molecules, and water are absorbed by the digestive epithelium. Compaction, Choice *C*, occurs when waste products are dehydrated and compacted. Ingestion, Choice *D*, is when food and liquids first enter the body through the mouth.

11. D: The gallbladder is the organ that is responsible for storing and concentrating bile before secreting it into the small intestine. The liver, Choice *A*, is responsible for producing bile. The pancreas, Choice *B*, is responsible for secreting digestive enzymes specific for different types of food. The stomach, Choice *C*, is where digestion occurs.

12. D: Cardiac muscle cells are involuntary and makes up the heart muscle, which pumps blood through the veins and arteries. Skeletal muscle, Choice *A*, helps with body movement by pulling on the bones of the skeleton. Smooth muscle, Choice *B*, is an involuntary, nonstriated muscle that is found in the digestive tract and other hollow internal organs, such as the urinary bladder and blood vessels. The intestines, Choice *C*, are made up of smooth muscle cells.

13. B: Neurons are responsible for transferring and processing information between the brain and other parts of the body. Neuroglia are cells that protect delicate neurons by making a frame around them. They also help to maintain a homeostatic environment around the neurons.

14. C: The autonomic nerve system is part of the efferent division of the peripheral nervous system (PNS). It controls involuntary muscles, such as smooth muscle and cardiac muscle, which are responsible for regulating heart rate, blood pressure, and body temperature. The central nervous system, Choice *A*, includes only the brain and the spinal cord. The somatic nervous system, Choice *B*, is also part of the efferent division of the PNS and controls voluntary skeletal muscle contractions, allowing for body movements. The afferent division of the PNS, Choice *D*, relays sensory information within the body.

15. A: The testes are the main reproductive organ of the male reproductive system. They are the gonads; they secrete androgens, and produce and store sperm cells. The prostate, vas deferens, and bulbourethral glands are all accessory organs of the male reproductive system. The prostate provides nourishment to sperm, the vas deferens transports sperm to the urethra, and the bulbourethral glands produce lubricating fluid for the urethra.

16. B: The ovaries produce only one mature gamete each month. If it is fertilized, the result is a zygote that develops into an embryo. The male reproductive system produces one-half billion sperm cells each day.

17. D: Once sperm enter the vagina, they travel through the uterus to the Fallopian tubes to fertilize a mature oocyte. The ovaries are responsible for producing the mature oocyte. The mammary glands produce nutrient-filled milk to nourish babies after birth.

18. C: The skin is the largest organ of the body, covering every external surface of the body and protecting the body's deeper tissues. The brain performs many complex functions, the large intestine is part of the gastrointestinal system, and the heart keeps blood pumping throughout the body, but none of these is largest organ in the body.

19. A: The skin has three major functions: protection, regulation, and sensation. It has a large supply of blood vessels that can dilate to allow heat loss when the body is too hot and constrict in order to retain heat when the body is cold. The organs of respiratory system are responsible for breathing and the mouth is responsible for ingestion.

20. B: The nails on a person's hands and feet provide a hard layer of protection over the soft skin underneath. The hair, Choice *A*, helps to protect against heat loss, provides sensation, and can filter air that enters the nose. The sweat glands, Choice *C*, help to regulate temperature. The sebaceous glands, Choice *D*, secrete sebum, which protects the skin from water loss and bacterial and fungal infections.

21. D: The tissues and glands of the endocrine system are all ductless. They secrete hormones, not bile, into the blood or interstitial fluid of the human body. The endocrine system has a slow, long-lasting response to stimuli, unlike the nervous system, whose response is quick and short termed.

22. A: The pituitary gland is a pea-sized gland that is found at the bottom of the hypothalamus. The hormones that it releases regulate growth, blood pressure, and pain relief, among other things. The thymus, Choice *B*, is located in the chest cavity and produces hormones that are important for the development and maintenance of immune responses. The thyroid gland, Choice *C*, is found in the neck and releases hormones responsible for metabolism, growth and development, temperature regulation, and brain development during infancy and childhood. The pancreas, Choice *D*, is located in the abdomen and regulates blood sugar levels.

23. C: The pancreas is responsible for regulating blood sugar levels in the body. The pineal gland regulates melatonin levels, which affect maturation of gametes and reproductive organs, as well as the body's circadian rhythm. The parathyroid gland secretes a hormone that helps the thyroid regulate calcium levels in the body. The adrenal glands help with the body's management of stress.

24. A: The kidneys are the main organs responsible for filtering waste products out of the bloodstream. The kidneys have millions of nephrons, which are tiny filtering units, that filter 120 to 150 quarts of blood each day and produce waste in the amount of approximately one to two quarts of urine daily. The urinary bladder is responsible for storage of urine. The pancreas is responsible for regulating blood sugar levels. The urethra is the passageway through which urine exits the body.

25. A: In the male genitourinary system, both urine and gametes travel through the urethra to exit the body. The sperm is produced by the testes and then travels through the urethra. Urine is produced by the kidneys, is stored in the urinary bladder, and then exits the body through the urethra. In females, the urethra is solely used for urine to exit the body. Gametes exit the body from the uterus and through the vagina.

26. C: The urinary bladder is a hollow, elastic muscular organ. As it fills with urine, the walls stretch without breaking—due to their elasticity—and become thinner. When the urine is emptied, the bladder returns to its original size. The urinary bladder does not secrete any fluids into the urine; it is a storage organ for urine. Pressure inside the urinary bladder does not increase as it is filled because the organ grows larger while filling.

27. A: The innate immune system works based on pattern recognition of similar pathogens that have already been encountered. It does not remember specific pathogens or provide an individually-specific response. The responses it provides are short term and do not work toward long-lasting immunity for the body. The adaptive immune system creates a memory of each specific pathogen that has been encountered and provides a pathogen-specific response. This works toward the long-term immunity of the body. Hormones are secreted by the endocrine system in response to stimuli. B cells are lymphocytes that work to provide immunity as part of the adaptive immune system.

28. B: The adaptive immune system provides target-specific antibodies to fight against individual pathogens that are encountered. It does not send out a broad range of antibodies because it has memory of the previously encountered pathogens. Mechanical and chemical barriers are part of the innate immune system and do not provide target-specific immunity.

29. D: If the immune system is not functioning properly, it may begin to attack its own healthy cells, which can result in an autoimmune disorder, such as celiac disease, type I diabetes, or rheumatoid arthritis. The adaptive and innate immune systems are the two parts of the body's immune system that need to be working properly to protect the body from pathogens. Lymphocytes are specialized cells that help the adaptive immune system provide target-specific responses to pathogens.

30. A: There are 206 bones in the adult human body. Human babies are born with three hundred bones. As they grow, bones fuse together and the body is left with 206 individual bones. There are twenty-seven bones in one human hand and twenty-six bones in one human foot.

31. D: Spongy bone is porous and lightweight, but also very strong. It covers the outside of dense, compact bone and has a shiny, white appearance. Compact bone is densely filled with organic and inorganic salts, leaving only tiny spaces for osteocytes within the matrix.

32. A: The skull, Choice *B*, is a set of bones that protect the brain. The ribs, Choice *C*, are a set of bones that protect the heart and lungs. The vertebrae, Choice *D*, are a set of bones that protect the spinal cord. The foot bones do not provide protection for delicate organs. They provide structure for the foot and support for the body.

33. A: Monosaccharides are the simplest sugars that make up carbohydrates. They are important for cellular respiration. Fatty acids, Choice *B*, make up lipids. Polysaccharides, Choice *C*, are larger molecules with repeating monosaccharide units. Amino acids, Choice *D*, are the building blocks of proteins.

34. D: Nucleic acids include DNA and RNA, which are strands of nucleotides that contain genetic information. Carbohydrates, Choice *A*, are made up of sugars that provide energy to the body. Lipids, Choice *B*, are hydrocarbon chains that make up fats. Proteins, Choice *C*, are made up of amino acids that help with many functions for maintaining life.

35. B: Genes are the primary unit of inheritance between generations of an organism. Humans each have twenty-three pairs of chromosomes (Choice *A*), and each chromosome contains hundreds to thousands of genes. Genes each control a specific trait of the organism. Gametes, Choice *C*, are the reproductive cells that contain all of the genetic information of an individual. Atoms, Choice *D*, are the small units that make up all substances.

36. C: The Law of Independent Assortment states that the alleles for different traits are inherited independently of one another. For example, the alleles for eye color are not linked to the alleles for hair color. So, someone could have blue eyes and brown hair or blue eyes and blond hair. The Law of Dominance, Choice *A*, states that one allele has a stronger effect on phenotype than the other allele. The Law of Segregation, Choice *B*, states that each trait has two versions that can be inherited. Each parent contributes one of its alleles, selected randomly, to the daughter offspring.

37. C: Atoms are considered neutral when the number of protons and electrons is equal. Protons carry a positive charge, and electrons carry a negative charge. When they are equal in number, their charges cancel out, and the atom is neutral. If there are more electrons than protons, or vice versa, the atom has an electric charge and is termed an ion. Neutrons do not have a charge and do not affect the electric charge of an atom.

38. A: Physical properties of substances are those that can be observed without changing the substances' chemical composition, such as odor, color, density, and hardness. Reactivity, flammability, and toxicity are all chemical properties of substances. They describe the way in which a substance may change into a different substance. They cannot be observed from the surface.

39. B: Solids have molecules that are packed together tightly and cannot move within their substance. Crystalline solids have atoms or molecules that are arranged symmetrically, making all of the bonds of even strength. When they are broken, they break along a plane of molecules, creating a straight edge. Amorphous solids do not have the symmetrical makeup of crystalline solids. They do not break evenly. Gases and liquids both have molecules that move around freely.

40. A: Chemical reactions are processes that involve the changing of one set of substances to a different set of substances. In order to accomplish this, the bonds between the atoms in the molecules of the original substances need to be broken. The atoms are rearranged, and new bonds are formed to make the new set of substances. Combination reactions involve two or more reactants becoming one product. Decomposition reactions involve one reactant becoming two or more products. Combustion reactions involve the use of oxygen as a reactant and generally include the burning of a substance. Choices *C* and *D* are not discussed as specific reaction types.

41. B: Newton meter. A Newton meter is used for such things such as gravity, friction, or tension. A bathroom scale or similar scale is a common example of a force meter. Choice *A* is not an existing term. Choices *C* and *D* are used to measure fractions of small numbers.

42. D: A Vernier Scale is used to measure small fractions within already small divisions. Choices *A*, *B*, and *C* are used for measuring short distances, yet do not go as small as the Vernier Scale.

43. D: Scientific experiments are found reliable when they can be replicated and produce comparable results regardless of who is conducting them or making the observations, making Choice *B* incorrect. Choice *A* is incorrect, although having all the materials needed is ideal for conducting an experiment. Choice *C* is incorrect; a hypothesis is never proven correct, but it can receive credibility if the data supports it in that particular experiment.

44. A: The drinking water being contaminated and the stomach cancer is not necessarily determined by cause and effect. The two events could have just happened at the same time, which is correlation, not causation. The other three examples are very clear examples of cause and effect; we know for a fact that when water becomes hot enough, it boils, or that earthquakes are caused by tectonic plates shifting.

45. C: Newton's Third Law. This law states that for every action, there is an opposite and equal reaction. When Camille pushes Harley forward on the swing, the opposite and equal reaction is the swing going backwards. Choice *A*, law of inertia, is Newton's first law, which states that an object at rest or at motion stays that way unless otherwise acted upon by an outside force, making Choice *A* incorrect. Choice *B*, Newton's second law, states that the heavier, an object, the more force has to be used to move it, making Choice *C* incorrect. Choice *D*, Law of Segregation, has to do with heredity, and states that each trait has two versions that can be inherited, making Choice *D* incorrect.

46. B: Formulating a hypothesis means writing out an expectation of what's going to happen. The hypothesis comes after the experimental question, which is forming a question that relates to the observation, making Choice *A* incorrect. Gathering the materials needed for the procedure is the step where we actually conduct the experiment, making Choice *C* incorrect. Summarizing the results of the experiment is the conclusion, making Choice *D* incorrect.

47. C: After the experiment is over and before it is published. A peer review is when other scientists review the experiment's findings in order to test its validity and methods. Peer review is an important part of scientific research and is a way for the scientific community to provide feedback for the experiment.

English and Language Usage

Conventions of Standard English

Conventions of Standard English Spelling

Homophones

Homophones are words that have different meanings and spellings, but sound the same. These can be confusing for English Language Learners (ELLs) and beginning students, but even native English-speaking adults can find them problematic unless informed by context. Whereas listeners must rely entirely on context to differentiate spoken homophone meanings, readers with good spelling knowledge have a distinct advantage since homophones are spelled differently. For instance, *their* means belonging to them; *there* indicates location; and *they're* is a contraction of *they are*; despite different meanings, they all sound the same. *Lacks* can be a plural noun or a present-tense, third-person singular verb; either way it refers to absence—*deficiencies* as a plural noun, and *is deficient in* as a verb. But *lax* is an adjective that means loose, slack, relaxed, uncontrolled, or negligent. These two spellings, derivations, and meanings are completely different. With speech, listeners cannot know spelling and must use context; but with print, readers with spelling knowledge can differentiate them with or without context.

Homonyms, Homophones, and Homographs

Homophones are words that sound the same in speech, but have different spellings and meanings. For example, *to, too,* and *two* all sound alike, but have three different spellings and meanings. Homophones with different spellings are also called heterographs. Homographs are words that are spelled identically, but have different meanings. If they also have different pronunciations, they are heteronyms. For instance, *tear* pronounced one way means a drop of liquid formed by the eye; pronounced another way, it means to rip. Homophones that are also homographs are homonyms. For example, *bark* can mean the outside of a tree or a dog's vocalization; both meanings have the same spelling. *Stalk* can mean a plant stem or to pursue and/or harass somebody; these are spelled and pronounced the same. *Rose* can mean a flower or the past tense of *rise*. Many non-linguists confuse things by using "homonym" to mean sets of words that are homophones but not homographs, and also those that are homographs but not homophones.

The word *row* can mean to use oars to propel a boat; a linear arrangement of objects or print; or an argument. It is pronounced the same with the first two meanings, but differently with the third. Because it is spelled identically regardless, all three meanings are homographs. However, the two meanings pronounced the same are homophones, whereas the one with the different pronunciation is a heteronym. By contrast, the word *read* means to peruse language, whereas the word *reed* refers to a marsh plant. Because these are pronounced the same way, they are homophones; because they are spelled differently, they are heterographs. Homonyms are both homophones and homographs—pronounced and spelled identically, but with different meanings. One distinction between homonyms is of those with separate, unrelated etymologies, called "true" homonyms, e.g. *skate* meaning a fish or *skate* meaning to glide over ice/water. Those with common origins are called polysemes or polysemous homonyms, e.g. the *mouth* of an animal/human or of a river.

Irregular Plurals

One type of irregular English plural involves words that are spelled the same whether they are singular or plural. These include *deer, fish, salmon, trout, sheep, moose, offspring, species, aircraft,* etc. The spelling rule for making these words plural is simple: they do not change. Another type of irregular English plurals does change from singular to plural form, but it does not take regular English –*s* or –*es* endings. Their irregular plural endings are largely derived from grammatical and spelling conventions in the other languages of their origins, like Latin, German, and vowel shifts and other linguistic mutations. Some examples of these words and their irregular plurals include *child* and *children; die* and *dice; foot* and *feet; goose* and *geese; louse* and *lice; man* and *men; mouse* and *mice; ox* and *oxen; person* and *people; tooth* and *teeth;* and *woman* and *women.*

Contractions

Contractions are formed by joining two words together, omitting one or more letters from one of the component words, and replacing the omitted words with an apostrophe. An obvious yet often forgotten rule for spelling contractions is to place the apostrophe where the letters were omitted; for example, spelling errors like *did'nt* for *didn't. Didn't* is a contraction of *did not.* Therefore, the apostrophe replaces the "o" that is omitted from the "not" component. Another common error is confusing contractions with possessives because both include apostrophes, e.g. spelling the possessive *its* as "it's," which is a contraction of "it is"; spelling the possessive *their* as "they're," a contraction of "they are"; spelling the possessive *whose* as "who's," a contraction of "who is"; or spelling the possessive *your* as "you're," a contraction of "you are."

Frequently Misspelled Words

One source of spelling errors is not knowing whether to drop the final letter *e* from a word when its form is changed by adding an ending to indicate the past tense or progressive participle of a verb, converting an adjective to an adverb, a noun to an adjective, etc. Some words retain the final *e* when another syllable is added; others lose it. For example, *true* becomes *truly; argue* becomes *arguing; come* becomes *coming; write* becomes *writing;* and *judge* becomes *judging.* In these examples, the final *e* is dropped before adding the ending. But *severe* becomes *severely; complete* becomes *completely; sincere* becomes *sincerely; argue* becomes *argued;* and *care* becomes *careful.* In these instances, the final *e* is retained before adding the ending. Note that some words, like *argue* in these examples, drops the final *e* when the *–ing* ending is added to indicate the participial form; but the regular past tense ending of *–ed* makes it *argued,* in effect replacing the final *e* so that *arguing* is spelled without an *e* but *argued* is spelled with one.

Some English words contain the vowel combination of *ei,* while some contain the reverse combination of *ie.* Many people confuse these. Some examples include these:

> *ceiling, conceive, leisure, receive, weird, their, either, foreign, sovereign, neither, neighbors, seize, forfeit, counterfeit, height, weight, protein,* and *freight*

Words with *ie* include *piece, believe, chief, field, friend, grief, relief, mischief, siege, niece, priest, fierce, pierce, achieve, retrieve, hygiene, science,* and *diesel.* A rule that also functions as a mnemonic device is "I before E except after C, or when sounded like A as in 'neighbor' or 'weigh'." However, it is obvious from the list above that many exceptions exist.

Many people often misspell certain words by confusing whether they have the vowel *a, e,* or *i,* frequently in the middle syllable of three-syllable words or beginning the last syllables that sound the same in different words. For example, in the following correctly spelled words, the vowel in boldface is the one people typically get wrong by substituting one or either of the others for it:

> cem**e**tery, quant**i**ties, ben**e**fit, privi**l**ege, unpleas**a**nt, sep**a**rate, independ**e**nt, excell**e**nt, cat**e**gories, indispens**a**ble, and irrelev**a**nt

The words with final syllables that sound the same when spoken but are spelled differently include *unpleasant, independent, excellent,* and *irrelevant.* Another source of misspelling is whether or not to double consonants when adding suffixes. For example, we double the last consonant before *–ed* and *–ing* endings in *controlled, beginning, forgetting, admitted, occurred, referred,* and *hopping;* but we do not double the last consonant before the suffix in *shining, poured, sweating, loving, hating, smiling,* and *hoping.*

One way in which people misspell certain words frequently is by failing to include letters that are silent. Some letters are articulated when pronounced correctly but elided in some people's speech, which then transfers to their writing. Another source of misspelling is the converse: people add extraneous letters. For example, some people omit the silent *u* in *guarantee,* overlook the first *r* in *surprise,* leave out the *z* in *realize,* fail to double the *m* in *recommend,* leave out the middle *i* from *aspirin,* and exclude the *p* from *temperature.* The converse error, adding extra letters, is common in words like *until* by adding a second *l* at the end; or by inserting a superfluous syllabic *a* or *e* in the middle of *athletic,* reproducing a common mispronunciation.

Conventions of Standard English Punctuation

Rules of Capitalization
The first word of any document, and of each new sentence, is capitalized. Proper nouns, like names and adjectives derived from proper nouns, should also be capitalized. Here are some examples:

- Grand Canyon
- Pacific Palisades
- Golden Gate Bridge
- Freudian slip
- Shakespearian, Spenserian, or Petrarchan sonnet
- Irish song

Some exceptions are adjectives, originally derived from proper nouns, which through time and usage are no longer capitalized, like *quixotic, herculean,* or *draconian.* Capitals draw attention to specific instances of people, places, and things. Some categories that should be capitalized include the following:

- brand names
- companies
- weekdays
- months
- governmental divisions or agencies
- historical eras
- major historical events
- holidays
- institutions
- famous buildings
- ships and other manmade constructions
- natural and manmade landmarks
- territories
- nicknames
- epithets
- organizations
- planets

- nationalities
- tribes
- religions
- names of religious deities
- roads
- special occasions, like the Cannes Film Festival or the Olympic Games

Exceptions

Related to American government, capitalize the noun Congress but not the related adjective congressional. Capitalize the noun U.S. Constitution, but not the related adjective constitutional. Many experts advise leaving the adjectives federal and state in lowercase, as in federal regulations or state water board, and only capitalizing these when they are parts of official titles or names, like Federal Communications Commission or State Water Resources Control Board. While the names of the other planets in the solar system are capitalized as names, Earth is more often capitalized only when being described specifically as a planet, like Earth's orbit, but lowercase otherwise since it is used not only as a proper noun but also to mean *land, ground, soil*, etc.

Names of animal species or breeds are not capitalized unless they include a proper noun. Then, only the proper noun is capitalized. Antelope, black bear, and yellow-bellied sapsucker are not capitalized. However, Bengal tiger, German shepherd, Australian shepherd, French poodle, and Russian blue cat are capitalized.

Other than planets, celestial bodies like the sun, moon, and stars are not capitalized. Medical conditions like tuberculosis or diabetes are lowercase; again, exceptions are proper nouns, like Epstein-Barr syndrome, Alzheimer's disease, and Down syndrome. Seasons and related terms like winter solstice or autumnal equinox are lowercase. Plants, including fruits and vegetables, like poinsettia, celery, or avocados, are not capitalized unless they include proper names, like Douglas fir, Jerusalem artichoke, Damson plums, or Golden Delicious apples.

Titles and Names

When official titles precede names, they should be capitalized, except when there is a comma between the title and name. But if a title follows or replaces a name, it should not be capitalized. For example, "the president" without a name is not capitalized, as in "The president addressed Congress." But with a name it is capitalized, like "President Obama addressed Congress." Or, "Chair of the Board Janet Yellen was appointed by President Obama." One exception is that some publishers and writers nevertheless capitalize President, Queen, Pope, etc., when these are not accompanied by names to show respect for these high offices. However, many writers in America object to this practice for violating democratic principles of equality. Occupations before full names are not capitalized, like owner Mark Cuban, director Martin Scorsese, or coach Roger McDowell.

Some universal rules for capitalization in composition titles include capitalizing the following:

- The first and last words of the title
- Forms of the verb *to be* and all other verbs
- Pronouns
- The word *not*

Universal rules for NOT capitalizing include the articles *the, a,* or *an;* the conjunctions *and, or,* or *nor,* and the preposition *to,* or *to* as part of the infinitive form of a verb. The exception to all of these is UNLESS any of them is the first or last word in the title, in which case they are capitalized. Other words are subject to differences of opinion and differences among various stylebooks or methods. These include *as, but, if,* and *or,* which some capitalize and others do not. Some authorities say no preposition should ever be capitalized; some say prepositions five or more letters long should be capitalized. The *Associated Press Stylebook* advises capitalizing prepositions longer than three letters (like *about, across,* or *with*).

Ellipses
Ellipses (. . .) signal omitted text when quoting. Some writers also use them to show a thought trailing off, but this should not be overused outside of dialogue. An example of an ellipses would be if someone is quoting a phrase out of a professional source but wants to omit part of the phrase that isn't needed: "Dr. Skim's analysis of pollen inside the body is clearly a myth . . . that speaks to the environmental guilt of our society."

Commas
Commas separate words or phrases in a series of three or more. The Oxford comma is the last comma in a series. Many people omit this last comma, but many times it causes confusion. Here is an example:

I love my sisters, the Queen of England and Madonna.

This example without the comma implies that the "Queen of England and Madonna" are the speaker's sisters. However, if the speaker was trying to say that they love their sisters, the Queen of England, as well as Madonna, there should be a comma after "Queen of England" to signify this.

Commas also separate two coordinate adjectives ("big, heavy dog") but not cumulative ones, which should be arranged in a particular order for them to make sense ("beautiful ancient ruins").

A comma ends the first of two independent clauses connected by conjunctions. Here is an example:

I ate a bowl of tomato soup, and I was hungry very shortly after.

Here are some brief rules for commas:

- Commas follow introductory words like *however, furthermore, well, why,* and *actually,* among others.
- Commas go between city and state: Houston, Texas.
- If using a comma between a surname and Jr. or Sr. or a degree like M.D., also follow the whole name with a comma: "Martin Luther King, Jr., wrote that."
- A comma follows a dependent clause beginning a sentence: "Although she was very small, . . ."
- Nonessential modifying words/phrases/clauses are enclosed by commas: "Wendy, who is Peter's sister, closed the window."
- Commas introduce or interrupt direct quotations: "She said, 'I hate him.' 'Why,' I asked, 'do you hate him?'"

Semicolons
Semicolons are used to connect two independent clauses, but should never be used in the place of a comma. They can replace periods between two closely connected sentences: "Call back tomorrow; it can wait until then." When writing items in a series and one or more of them contains internal commas, separate them with semicolons, like the following:

People came from Springfield, Illinois; Alamo, Tennessee; Moscow, Idaho; and other locations.

Hyphens

Here are some rules concerning hyphens:

- Compound adjectives like state-of-the-art or off-campus are hyphenated.
- Original compound verbs and nouns are often hyphenated, like "throne-sat," "video-gamed," "no-meater."
- Adjectives ending in –ly are often hyphenated, like "family-owned" or "friendly-looking."
- "Five years old" is not hyphenated, but singular ages like "five-year-old" are.
- Hyphens can clarify. For example, in "stolen vehicle report," "stolen-vehicle report" clarifies that "stolen" modifies "vehicle," not "report."
- Compound numbers twenty-one through ninety-nine are spelled with hyphens.
- Prefixes before proper nouns/adjectives are hyphenated, like "mid-September" and "trans-Pacific."

Parentheses

Parentheses enclose information such as an aside or more clarifying information: "She ultimately replied (after deliberating for an hour) that she was undecided." They are also used to insert short, in-text definitions or acronyms: "His FBS (fasting blood sugar) was higher than normal." When parenthetical information ends the sentence, the period follows the parentheses: "We received new funds ($25,000)." Only put periods within parentheses if the whole sentence is inside them: "Look at this. (You'll be astonished.)" However, this can also be acceptable as a clause: "Look at this (you'll be astonished)." Although parentheses appear to be part of the sentence subject, they are not, and do not change subject-verb agreement: "Will (and his dog) was there."

Quotation Marks

Quotation marks are typically used when someone is quoting a direct word or phrase someone else writes or says. Additionally, quotation marks should be used for the titles of poems, short stories, songs, articles, chapters, and other shorter works. When quotations include punctuation, periods and commas should *always* be placed inside of the quotation marks.

When a quotation contains another quotation inside of it, the outer quotation should be enclosed in double quotation marks and the inner quotation should be enclosed in single quotation marks. For example: "Timmy was begging, 'Don't go! Don't leave!'" When using both double and single quotation marks, writers will find that many word-processing programs may automatically insert enough space between the single and double quotation marks to be visible for clearer reading. But if this is not the case, the writer should write/type them with enough space between to keep them from looking like three single quotation marks. Additionally, non-standard usages, terms used in an unusual fashion, and technical terms are often clarified by quotation marks. Here are some examples:

My "friend," Dr. Sims, has been micromanaging me again.

This way of extracting oil has been dubbed "fracking."

Apostrophes

One use of the apostrophe is followed by an *s* to indicate possession, like *Mrs. White's home* or *our neighbor's dog*. When using the *'s* after names or nouns that also end in the letter *s*, no single rule applies: some experts advise adding both the apostrophe and the *s*, like "the Jones's house," while others prefer using only the apostrophe and omitting the additional *s*, like "the Jones' house." The wisest expert advice is to pick one formula or the other and then apply it consistently. Newspapers and magazines often use *'s* after common nouns ending with *s*, but add only the apostrophe after proper nouns or names ending with *s*. One common error is to place the apostrophe before a name's final *s* instead of after it: "Ms. Hasting's book" is incorrect if the name is Ms. Hastings.

Plural nouns should not include apostrophes (e.g. "apostrophe's"). Exceptions are to clarify atypical plurals, like verbs used as nouns: "These are the do's and don'ts." Irregular plurals that do not end in *s* always take apostrophe-*s*, not *s*-apostrophe—a common error, as in "childrens' toys," which should be "children's toys." Compound nouns like mother-in-law, when they are singular and possessive, are followed by apostrophe-*s*, like "your mother-in-law's coat." When a compound noun is plural and possessive, the plural is formed before the apostrophe-*s*, like "your sisters-in-laws' coats." When two people named possess the same thing, use apostrophe-*s* after the second name only, like "Dennis and Pam's house."

Sentence Structures

Incomplete Sentences

Four types of incomplete sentences are sentence fragments, run-on sentences, subject-verb and/or pronoun-antecedent disagreement, and non-parallel structure.

Sentence fragments are caused by absent subjects, absent verbs, or dangling/uncompleted dependent clauses. Every sentence must have a subject and a verb to be complete. An example of a fragment is "Raining all night long," because there is no subject present. "It was raining all night long" is one correction. Another example of a sentence fragment is the second part in "Many scientists think in unusual ways. Einstein, for instance." The second phrase is a fragment because it has no verb. One correction is "Many scientists, like Einstein, think in unusual ways." Finally, look for "cliffhanger" words like *if, when, because,* or *although* that introduce dependent clauses, which cannot stand alone without an independent clause. For example, to correct the sentence fragment "If you get home early," add an independent clause: "If you get home early, we can go dancing."

Run-On Sentences

A run-on sentence combines two or more complete sentences without punctuating them correctly or separating them. For example, a run-on sentence caused by a lack of punctuation is the following:

> There is a malfunction in the computer system however there is nobody available right now who knows how to troubleshoot it.

One correction is, "There is a malfunction in the computer system; however, there is nobody available right now who knows how to troubleshoot it." Another is, "There is a malfunction in the computer system. However, there is nobody available right now who knows how to troubleshoot it."

An example of a comma splice of two sentences is the following:

> Jim decided not to take the bus, he walked home.

Replacing the comma with a period or a semicolon corrects this. Commas that try and separate two independent clauses without a contraction are considered comma splices.

Parallel Sentence Structures

Parallel structure in a sentence matches the forms of sentence components. Any sentence containing more than one description or phrase should keep them consistent in wording and form. Readers can easily follow writers' ideas when they are written in parallel structure, making it an important element of correct sentence construction. For example, this sentence lacks parallelism: "Our coach is a skilled manager, a clever strategist, and works hard." The first two phrases are parallel, but the third is not. Correction: "Our coach is a skilled manager, a clever strategist, and a hard worker." Now all three phrases match in form. Here is another example:

Fred intercepted the ball, escaped tacklers, and a touchdown was scored.

This is also non-parallel. Here is the sentence corrected:

Fred intercepted the ball, escaped tacklers, and scored a touchdown.

Sentence Fluency
For fluent composition, writers must use a variety of sentence types and structures, and also ensure that they smoothly flow together when they are read. To accomplish this, they must first be able to identify fluent writing when they read it. This includes being able to distinguish among simple, compound, complex, and compound-complex sentences in text; to observe variations among sentence types, lengths, and beginnings; and to notice figurative language and understand how it augments sentence length and imparts musicality. Once students/writers recognize superior fluency, they should revise their own writing to be more readable and fluent. They must be able to apply acquired skills to revisions before being able to apply them to new drafts.

One strategy for revising writing to increase its sentence fluency is flipping sentences. This involves rearranging the word order in a sentence without deleting, changing, or adding any words. For example, the student or other writer who has written the sentence, "We went bicycling on Saturday" can revise it to, "On Saturday, we went bicycling." Another technique is using appositives. An appositive is a phrase or word that renames or identifies another adjacent word or phrase. Writers can revise for sentence fluency by inserting main phrases/words from one shorter sentence into another shorter sentence, combining them into one longer sentence, e.g. from "My cat Peanut is a gray and brown tabby. He loves hunting rats." to "My cat Peanut, a gray and brown tabby, loves hunting rats." Revisions can also connect shorter sentences by using conjunctions and commas and removing repeated words: "Scott likes eggs. Scott is allergic to eggs" becomes "Scott likes eggs, but he is allergic to them."

One technique for revising writing to increase sentence fluency is "padding" short, simple sentences by adding phrases that provide more details specifying why, how, when, and/or where something took place. For example, a writer might have these two simple sentences: "I went to the market. I purchased a cake." To revise these, the writer can add the following informative dependent and independent clauses and prepositional phrases, respectively: "Before my mother woke up, I sneaked out of the house and went to the supermarket. As a birthday surprise, I purchased a cake for her." When revising sentences to make them longer, writers must also punctuate them correctly to change them from simple sentences to compound, complex, or compound-complex sentences.

Skills Writers Can Employ to Increase Fluency
One way writers can increase fluency is by varying the beginnings of sentences. Writers do this by starting most of their sentences with different words and phrases rather than monotonously repeating the same ones across multiple sentences. Another way writers can increase fluency is by varying the lengths of sentences. Since run-on sentences are incorrect, writers make sentences longer by also converting them from simple to compound, complex, and compound-complex sentences. The coordination and subordination involved in these also give the text more variation and interest, hence more fluency.

Here are a few more ways writers can increase fluency:

- Varying the transitional language and conjunctions used makes sentences more fluent.
- Writing sentences with a variety of rhythms by using prepositional phrases.
- Varying sentence structure adds fluency.

Knowledge of Language

Use Grammar to Enhance Clarity in Writing

Possessives

Possessive forms indicate possession, i.e. that something belongs to or is owned by someone or something. As such, the most common parts of speech to be used in possessive form are adjectives, nouns, and pronouns. The rule for correctly spelling/punctuating possessive nouns and proper nouns is with - *'s,* like "the woman's briefcase" or "Frank's hat." With possessive adjectives, however, apostrophes are not used: these include *my, your, his, her, its, our,* and *their,* like "my book," "your friend," "his car," "her house," "its contents," "our family," or "their property." Possessive pronouns include *mine, yours, his, hers, its, ours,* and *theirs.* These also have no apostrophes. The difference is that possessive adjectives take direct objects, whereas possessive pronouns replace them. For example, instead of using two possessive adjectives in a row, as in "I forgot my book, so Blanca let me use her book," which reads monotonously, replacing the second one with a possessive pronoun reads better: "I forgot my book, so Blanca let me use hers."

Pronouns

There are three pronoun cases: subjective case, objective case, and possessive case. Pronouns as subjects are pronouns that replace the subject of the sentence, such as *I, you, he, she, it, we, they* and *who.* Pronouns as objects replace the object of the sentence, such as *me, you, him, her, it, us, them,* and *whom.* Pronouns that show possession are *mine, yours, hers, its, ours, theirs,* and *whose.* The following are examples of different pronoun cases:

- Subject pronoun: *She* ate the cake for her birthday. *I* saw the movie.
- Object pronoun: You gave *me* the card last weekend. She gave the picture to *him.*
- Possessive pronoun: That bracelet you found yesterday is *mine. His* name was Casey.

Adjectives

Adjectives are descriptive words that modify nouns or pronouns. They may occur before or after the nouns or pronouns they modify in sentences. For example, in "This is a big house," *big* is an adjective modifying or describing the noun *house.* In "This house is big," the adjective is at the end of the sentence rather than preceding the noun it modifies.

A rule of punctuation that applies to adjectives is to separate a series of adjectives with commas. For example, "Their home was a large, rambling, old, white, two-story house." A comma should never separate the last adjective from the noun, though.

Adverbs

Whereas adjectives modify and describe nouns or pronouns, adverbs modify and describe adjectives, verbs, or other adverbs. Adverbs can be thought of as answers to questions in that they describe when, where, how, how often, how much, or to what extent.

Many (but not all) adjectives can be converted to adverbs by adding –*ly*. For example, in "She is a quick learner," *quick* is an adjective modifying *learner*. In "She learns quickly," *quickly* is an adverb modifying *learns*. One exception is *fast*. *Fast* is an adjective in "She is a fast learner." However, –*ly* is never added to the word *fast*; it retains the same form as an adverb in "She learns fast."

Verbs

A verb is a word or phrase that expresses action, feeling, or state of being. Verbs explain what their subject is *doing*. Three different types of verbs used in a sentence are action verbs, linking verbs, and helping verbs.

Action verbs show a physical or mental action. Some examples of action verbs are *play, type, jump, write, examine, study, invent, develop,* and *taste*. The following example uses an action verb:

> Kat *imagines* that she is a mermaid in the ocean.

The verb *imagines* explains what Kat is doing: she is imagining being a mermaid.

Linking verbs connect the subject to the predicate without expressing an action. The following sentence shows an example of a linking verb:

> The mango *tastes* sweet.

The verb *tastes* is a linking verb. The mango doesn't *do* the tasting, but the word *taste* links the mango to its predicate, sweet. Most linking verbs can also be used as action verbs, such as *smell, taste, look, seem, grow,* and *sound*. Saying something *is* something else is also an example of a linking verb. For example, if we were to say, "Peaches is a dog," the verb *is* would be a linking verb in this sentence, since it links the subject to its predicate.

Helping verbs are verbs that help the main verb in a sentence. Examples of helping verbs are *be, am, is, was, have, has, do, did, can, could, may, might, should,* and *must*, among others. The following are examples of helping verbs:

> Jessica *is* planning a trip to Hawaii.
>
> Brenda *does* not like camping.
>
> Xavier *should* go to the dance tonight.

Notice that after each of these helping verbs is the main verb of the sentence: *planning, like,* and *go*. Helping verbs usually show an aspect of time.

Transitional Words and Phrases

In connected writing, some sentences naturally lead to others, whereas in other cases, a new sentence expresses a new idea. We use transitional phrases to connect sentences and the ideas they convey. This makes the writing coherent. Transitional language also guides the reader from one thought to the next. For example, when pointing out an objection to the previous idea, starting a sentence with "However," "But," or "On the other hand" is transitional. When adding another idea or detail, writers use "Also," "In addition," "Furthermore," "Further," "Moreover," "Not only," etc. Readers have difficulty perceiving connections between ideas without such transitional wording.

Subject-Verb Agreement

Lack of subject-verb agreement is a very common grammatical error. One of the most common instances is when people use a series of nouns as a compound subject with a singular instead of a plural verb. Here is an example:

> Identifying the best books, locating the sellers with the lowest prices, and paying for them *is* difficult

instead of saying "*are* difficult." Additionally, when a sentence subject is compound, the verb is plural:

> He and his cousins *were* at the reunion.

However, if the conjunction connecting two or more singular nouns or pronouns is "or" or "nor," the verb must be singular to agree:

> That pen or another one like it is in the desk drawer.

If a compound subject includes both a singular noun and a plural one, and they are connected by "or" or "nor," the verb must agree with the subject closest to the verb: "Sally or her sisters go jogging daily"; but "Her sisters or Sally goes jogging daily."

Simply put, singular subjects require singular verbs and plural subjects require plural verbs. A common source of agreement errors is not identifying the sentence subject correctly. For example, people often write sentences incorrectly like, "The group of students *were* complaining about the test." The subject is not the plural "students" but the singular "group." Therefore, the correct sentence should read, "The group of students *was* complaining about the test." The converse also applies, for example, in this incorrect sentence: "The facts in that complicated court case *is* open to question." The subject of the sentence is not the singular "case" but the plural "facts." Hence the sentence would correctly be written: "The facts in that complicated court case *are* open to question." New writers should not be misled by the distance between the subject and verb, especially when another noun with a different number intervenes as in these examples. The verb must agree with the subject, not the noun closest to it.

Pronoun-Antecedent Agreement

Pronouns within a sentence must refer specifically to one noun, known as the **antecedent.** Sometimes, if there are multiple nouns within a sentence, it may be difficult to ascertain which noun belongs to the pronoun. It's important that the pronouns always clearly reference the nouns in the sentence so as not to confuse the reader. Here's an example of an unclear pronoun reference:

> After Catherine cut Libby's hair, David bought her some lunch.

The pronoun in the examples above is *her*. The pronoun could either be referring to *Catherine* or *Libby*. Here are some ways to write the above sentence with a clear pronoun reference:

> After Catherine cut Libby's hair, David bought Libby some lunch.

> David bought Libby some lunch after Catherine cut Libby's hair.

But many times the pronoun will clearly refer to its antecedent, like the following:

> After David cut Catherine's hair, he bought her some lunch.

Formal and Informal Language

Formal language is less personal than informal language. It is more "buttoned-up" and business-like, adhering to proper grammatical rules. It is used in professional or academic contexts, to convey respect or authority. For example, one would use formal language to write an informative or argumentative essay for school or to address a superior. Formal language avoids contractions, slang, colloquialisms, and first-person pronouns. Formal language uses sentences that are usually more complex and often in passive voice. Punctuation can differ as well. For example, exclamation points (!) are used to show strong emotion or can be used as an interjection but should be used sparingly in formal writing situations.

Informal language is often used when communicating with family members, friends, peers, and those known more personally. It is more casual, spontaneous, and forgiving in its conformity to grammatical rules and conventions. Informal language is used for personal emails and correspondence between coworkers or other familial relationships. The tone is more relaxed. In informal writing, slang, contractions, clichés, and the first- and second-person are often used.

Elements of the Writing Process

Skilled writers undergo a series of steps that comprise the writing process. The purpose of adhering to a structured approach to writing is to develop clear, meaningful, coherent work.

The stages are pre-writing or planning, organizing, drafting/writing, revising, and editing. Not every writer will necessarily follow all five stages for every project, but will judiciously employ the crucial components of the stages for most formal or important work. For example, a brief informal response to a short reading passage may not necessitate the need for significant organization after idea generation, but larger assignments and essays will likely mandate use of the full process.

Pre-Writing/Planning
Brainstorming
One of the most important steps in writing is pre-writing. Before drafting an essay or other assignment, it's helpful to think about the topic for a moment or two, in order to gain a more solid understanding of what the task is. Then, spend about five minutes jotting down the immediate ideas that could work for the essay. Brainstorming is a way to get some words on the page and offer a reference for ideas when drafting. Scratch paper is provided for writers to use any pre-writing techniques such as webbing, freewriting, or listing. Some writers prefer using graphic organizers during this phase. The goal is to get ideas out of the mind and onto the page.

Freewriting
Like brainstorming, freewriting is another prewriting activity to help the writer generate ideas. This method involves setting a timer for two or three minutes and writing down all ideas that come to mind about the topic using complete sentences. Once time is up, writers should review the sentences to see what observations have been made and how these ideas might translate into a more unified direction for the topic. Even if sentences lack sense as a whole, freewriting is an excellent way to get ideas onto the page in the very beginning stages of writing. Using complete sentences can make this a bit more challenging than brainstorming, but overall it is a worthwhile exercise, as it may force the writer to come up with more complete thoughts about the topic.

Once the ideas are on the page, it's time for the writer to turn them into a solid plan for the essay. The best ideas from the brainstorming results can then be developed into a more formal outline.

Organizing

Although sometimes it is difficult to get going on the brainstorming or prewriting phase, once ideas start flowing, writers often find that they have amassed too many thoughts that will not make for a cohesive and unified essay. During the organization stage, writers should examine the generated ideas, hone in on the important ones central to their main idea, and arrange the points in a logical and effective manner. Writers may also determine that some of the ideas generated in the planning process need further elaboration, potentially necessitating the need for research to gather infortmation to fill the gaps.

Once a writer has chosen his or her thesis and main argument, selected the most applicable details and evidence, and eliminated the "clutter," it is time to strategically organize the ideas. This is often accomplished with an outline.

Outlining

An **outline** is a system used to organize writing. When composing essays, outlining is important because it helps writers organize important information in a logical pattern using Roman numerals. Usually, outlines start out with the main ideas and then branch out into subgroups or subsidiary thoughts or subjects. Not only do outlines provide a visual tool for writers to reflect on how events, ideas, evidence, or other key parts of the argument relate to one another, but they can also lead writers to a stronger conclusion. The sample below demonstrates what a general outline looks like:

I. Introduction
      1. Background
      2. Thesis statement
II. Body
      1. Point A
          a. Supporting evidence
          b. Supporting evidence
      2. Point B
          a. Supporting evidence
          b. Supporting evidence
      3. Point C
          a. Supporting evidence
          b. Supporting evidence
III. Conclusion
      1. Restate main points of the paper.
      2. End with something memorable.

Drafting/Writing

Now it comes time to actually write the essay. In this stage, writers should follow the outline they developed in the brainstorming process and try to incorporate the useful sentences penned in the freewriting exercise. The main goal of this phase is to put all the thoughts together in cohesive sentences and paragraphs.

It is helpful for writers to remember that their work here does not have to be perfect. This process is often referred to as **drafting** because writers are just creating a rough draft of their work. Because of this, writers should avoid getting bogged down on the small details.

Referencing Sources

Anytime a writer quotes or paraphrases another text, they will need to include a citation. A **citation** is a short description of the work that a quote or information came from. The style manual your teacher wants you to follow will dictate exactly how to format that citation. For example, this is how one would cite a book according to the APA manual of style:

- *Format:* Last name, First initial, Middle initial. (Year Published) *Book Title.* City, State: Publisher.
- *Example:* Sampson, M. R. (1989). *Diaries from an Alien Invasion. Springfield, IL:* Campbell Press.

Revising

Revising offers an opportunity for writers to polish things up. Putting one's self in the reader's shoes and focusing on what the essay actually says helps writers identify problems—it's a movement from the mindset of writer to the mindset of editor. The goal is to have a clean, clear copy of the essay.

The main goal of the revision phase is to improve the essay's flow, cohesiveness, readability, and focus. For example, an essay will make a less persuasive argument if the various pieces of evidence are scattered and presented illogically or clouded with unnecessary thought. Therefore, writers should consider their essay's structure and organization, ensuring that there are smooth transitions between sentences and paragraphs. There should be a discernable introduction and conclusion as well, as these crucial components of an essay provide readers with a blueprint to follow.

Additionally, if the writer includes copious details that do little to enhance the argument, they may actually distract readers from focusing on the main ideas and detract from the strength of their work. The ultimate goal is to retain the purpose or focus of the essay and provide a reader-friendly experience. Because of this, writers often need to delete parts of their essay to improve its flow and focus. Removing sentences, entire paragraphs, or large chunks of writing can be one of the toughest parts of the writing process because it is difficult to part with work one has done. However, ultimately, these types of cuts can significantly improve one's essay.

Lastly, writers should consider their voice and word choice. The voice should be consistent throughout and maintain a balance between an authoritative and warm style, to both inform and engage readers. One way to alter voice is through word choice. Writers should consider changing weak verbs to stronger ones and selecting more precise language in areas where wording is vague. In some cases, it is useful to modify sentence beginnings or to combine or split up sentences to provide a more varied sentence structure.

Editing

Rather than focusing on content (as is the aim in the revising stage), the editing phase is all about the mechanics of the essay: the syntax, word choice, and grammar. This can be considered the proofreading stage. Successful editing is what sets apart a messy essay from a polished document.

The following areas should be considered when proofreading:

- Sentence fragments
- Awkward sentence structure
- Run-on sentences
- Incorrect word choice
- Grammatical agreement errors
- Spelling errors
- Punctuation errors
- Capitalization errors

One of the most effective ways of identifying grammatical errors, awkward phrases, or unclear sentences is to read the essay out loud. Listening to one's own work can help move the writer from simply the author to the reader.

During the editing phase, it's also important to ensure the essay follows the correct formatting and citation rules as dictated by the assignment.

Recursive Writing Process
While the writing process may have specific steps, the good news is that the process is recursive, meaning the steps need not be completed in a particular order. Many writers find that they complete steps at the same time such as drafting and revising, where the writing and rearranging of ideas occur simultaneously or in very close order. Similarly, a writer may find that a particular section of a draft needs more development, and will go back to the prewriting stage to generate new ideas. The steps can be repeated at any time, and the more these steps of the recursive writing process are employed, the better the final product will be.

Practice Makes Prepared Writers
Like any other useful skill, writing only improves with practice. While writing may come more easily to some than others, it is still a skill to be honed and improved. Regardless of a person's natural abilities, there is always room for growth in writing. Practicing the basic skills of writing can aid in preparations for the TEAS.

One way to build vocabulary and enhance exposure to the written word is through reading. This can be through reading books, but reading of any materials such as newspapers, magazines, and even social media count towards practice with the written word. This also helps to enhance critical reading and thinking skills, through analysis of the ideas and concepts read. Think of each new reading experience as a chance to sharpen these skills.

Developing a Well-Organized Paragraph

A **paragraph** is a series of connected and related sentences addressing one topic. Writing good paragraphs benefits writers by helping them to stay on target while drafting and revising their work. It benefits readers by helping them to follow the writing more easily. Regardless of how brilliant their ideas may be, writers who do not present them in organized ways will fail to engage readers—and fail to accomplish their writing goals. A fundamental rule for paragraphing is to confine each paragraph to a single idea. When writers find themselves transitioning to a new idea, they should start a new paragraph. However, a paragraph can include several pieces of evidence supporting its single idea; and it can include several points if they are all related to the overall paragraph topic. When writers find each point becoming lengthy, they may choose instead to devote a separate paragraph to every point and elaborate upon each more fully.

An effective paragraph should have these elements:

- Unity: One major discussion point or focus should occupy the whole paragraph from beginning to end.

- Coherence: For readers to understand a paragraph, it must be coherent. Two components of coherence are logical and verbal bridges. In logical bridges, the writer may write consecutive sentences with parallel structure or carry an idea over across sentences. In verbal bridges, writers may repeat key words across sentences.

- A topic sentence: The paragraph should have a sentence that generally identifies the paragraph's thesis or main idea.

- Sufficient development: To develop a paragraph, writers can use the following techniques after stating their topic sentence:

   o Define terms
   o Cite data
   o Use illustrations, anecdotes, and examples
   o Evaluate causes and effects
   o Analyze the topic
   o Explain the topic using chronological order

A **topic sentence** identifies the main idea of the paragraph. Some are explicit, some implicit. The topic sentence can appear anywhere in the paragraph. However, many experts advise beginning writers to place each paragraph topic sentence at or near the beginning of its paragraph to ensure that their readers understand what the topic of each paragraph is. Even without having written an explicit topic sentence, the writer should still be able to summarize readily what subject matter each paragraph addresses. The writer must then fully develop the topic that is introduced or identified in the topic sentence. Depending on what the writer's purpose is, they may use different methods for developing each paragraph.

Two main steps in the process of organizing paragraphs and essays should both be completed after determining the writing's main point, while the writer is planning or outlining the work. The initial step is to give an order to the topics addressed in each paragraph. Writers must have logical reasons for putting one paragraph first, another second, etc. The second step is to sequence the sentences in each paragraph. As with the first step, writers must have logical reasons for the order of sentences. Sometimes the work's main point obviously indicates a specific order.

Topic Sentences
To be effective, a topic sentence should be concise so that readers get its point without losing the meaning among too many words. As an example, in *Only Yesterday: An Informal History of the 1920s* (1931), author Frederick Lewis Allen's topic sentence introduces his paragraph describing the 1929 stock market crash: "The Bull Market was dead." This example illustrates the criteria of conciseness and brevity. It is also a strong sentence, expressed clearly and unambiguously. The topic sentence also introduces the paragraph, alerting the reader's attention to the main idea of the paragraph and the subject matter that follows the topic sentence.

Experts often recommend opening a paragraph with the topic sentences to enable the reader to realize the main point of the paragraph immediately. Application letters for jobs and university admissions also benefit from opening with topic sentences. However, positioning the topic sentence at the end of a paragraph is more logical when the paragraph identifies a number of specific details that accumulate evidence and then culminates with a generalization. While paragraphs with extremely obvious main ideas need no topic sentences, more often—and particularly for students learning to write—the topic sentence is the most important sentence in the paragraph. It not only communicates the main idea quickly to readers; it also helps writers produce and control information.

Vocabulary Acquisition

Context Clues

Readers can often figure out what unfamiliar words mean without interrupting their reading to look them up in dictionaries by examining context. **Context** includes the other words or sentences in a passage. One common context clue is the root word and any affixes (prefixes/suffixes). Another common context clue is a synonym or definition included in the sentence. Sometimes both exist in the same sentence. Here's an example:

> Scientists who study birds are *ornithologists*.

Many readers may not know the word *ornithologist*. However, the example contains a definition (scientists who study birds). The reader may also have the ability to analyze the suffix (*-logy*, meaning the study of) and root (*ornitho-*, meaning bird).

Another common context clue is a sentence that shows differences. Here's an example:

> Birds *incubate* their eggs outside of their bodies, unlike mammals.

Some readers may be unfamiliar with the word *incubate*. However, since we know that "unlike mammals," birds incubate their eggs outside of their bodies, we can infer that *incubate* has something to do with keeping eggs warm outside the body until they are hatched.

In addition to analyzing the etymology of a word's root and affixes and extrapolating word meaning from sentences that contrast an unknown word with an antonym, readers can also determine word meanings from sentence context clues based on logic. Here's an example:

> Birds are always looking out for predators that could attack their young.

The reader who is unfamiliar with the word *predator* could determine from the context of the sentence that predators usually prey upon baby birds and possibly other young animals. Readers might also use the context clue of etymology here, as *predator* and *prey* have the same root.

Analyzing Word Parts

By learning some of the etymologies of words and their parts, readers can break new words down into components and analyze their combined meanings. For example, the root word *soph* is Greek for wise or knowledge. Knowing this informs the meanings of English words including *sophomore, sophisticated,* and *philosophy*. Those who also know that *phil* is Greek for love will realize that *philosophy* means the love of knowledge. They can then extend this knowledge of *phil* to understand *philanthropist* (one who loves people), *bibliophile* (book lover), *philharmonic* (loving harmony), *hydrophilic* (water-loving), and so on. In addition, *phob-* derives from the Greek *phobos*, meaning fear. This informs all words ending with it as meaning fear of various things: *acrophobia* (fear of heights), *arachnophobia* (fear of spiders), *claustrophobia* (fear of enclosed spaces), *ergophobia* (fear of work), and *hydrophobia* (fear of water), among others.

Some English word origins from other languages, like ancient Greek, are found in large numbers and varieties of English words. An advantage of the shared ancestry of these words is that once readers recognize the meanings of some Greek words or word roots, they can determine or at least get an idea of what many different English words mean. As an example, the Greek word *métron* means to measure, a measure, or something used to measure; the English word meter derives from it. Knowing this informs many other English words, including *altimeter, barometer, diameter, hexameter, isometric,* and *metric.* While readers must know the meanings of the other parts of these words to decipher their meaning fully, they already have an idea that they are all related in some way to measures or measuring.

While all English words ultimately derive from a proto-language known as Indo-European, many of them historically came into the developing English vocabulary later, from sources like the ancient Greeks' language, the Latin used throughout Europe and much of the Middle East during the reign of the Roman Empire, and the Anglo-Saxon languages used by England's early tribes. In addition to classic revivals and native foundations, by the Renaissance era other influences included French, German, Italian, and Spanish. Today we can often discern English word meanings by knowing common roots and affixes, particularly from Greek and Latin.

The following is a list of common prefixes and their meanings:

Prefix	Definition	Examples
a-	Without	atheist, agnostic
ad-	to, toward	advance
ante-	Before	antecedent, antedate
anti-	Opposing	antipathy, antidote
auto-	Self	autonomy, autobiography
bene-	well, good	benefit, benefactor
bi-	Two	bisect, biennial
bio-	Life	biology, biosphere
chron-	Time	chronometer, synchronize
circum-	Around	circumspect, circumference
com-	with, together	commotion, complicate
contra-	against, opposing	contradict, contravene
cred-	belief, trust	credible, credit
de-	From	depart
dem-	People	demographics, democracy
dis-	away, off, down, not	dissent, disappear
equi-	equal, equally	equivalent
ex-	former, out of	extract
for-	away, off, from	forget, forswear
fore-	before, previous	foretell, forefathers
homo-	same, equal	homogenized
hyper-	excessive, over	hypercritical, hypertension
in-	in, into	intrude, invade
inter-	among, between	intercede, interrupt
mal-	bad, poorly, not	malfunction
micr-	Small	microbe, microscope
mis-	bad, poorly, not	misspell, misfire
mono-	one, single	monogamy, monologue
mor-	die, death	mortality, mortuary
neo-	New	neolithic, neoconservative

non-	not	nonentity, nonsense
omni-	all, everywhere	omniscient
over-	above	overbearing
pan-	all, entire	panorama, pandemonium
para-	beside, beyond	parallel, paradox
phil-	love, affection	philosophy, philanthropic
poly-	many	polymorphous, polygamous
pre-	before, previous	prevent, preclude
prim-	first, early	primitive, primary
pro-	forward, in place of	propel, pronoun
re-	back, backward, again	revoke, recur
sub-	under, beneath	subjugate, substitute
super-	above, extra	supersede, supernumerary
trans-	across, beyond, over	transact, transport
ultra-	beyond, excessively	ultramodern, ultrasonic, ultraviolet
un-	not, reverse of	unhappy, unlock
vis-	to see	visage, visible

The following is a list of common suffixes and their meanings:

Suffix	Definition	Examples
-able	likely, able to	capable, tolerable
-ance	act, condition	acceptance, vigilance
-ard	one that does excessively	drunkard, wizard
-ation	action, state	occupation, starvation
-cy	state, condition	accuracy, captaincy
-er	one who does	teacher
-esce	become, grow, continue	convalesce, acquiesce
-esque	in the style of, like	picturesque, grotesque
-ess	feminine	waitress, lioness
-ful	full of, marked by	thankful, zestful
-ible	able, fit	edible, possible, divisible
-ion	action, result, state	union, fusion
-ish	suggesting, like	churlish, childish
-ism	act, manner, doctrine	barbarism, socialism
-ist	doer, believer	monopolist, socialist
-ition	action, result, state,	sedition, expedition
-ity	quality, condition	acidity, civility
-ize	cause to be, treat with	sterilize, mechanize, criticize
-less	lacking, without	hopeless, countless
-like	like, similar	childlike, dreamlike
-ly	like, of the nature of	friendly, positively
-ment	means, result, action	refreshment, disappointment
-ness	quality, state	greatness, tallness
-or	doer, office, action	juror, elevator, honor
-ous	marked by, given to	religious, riotous

-some	apt to, showing	tiresome, lonesome
-th	act, state, quality	warmth, width
-ty	quality, state	enmity, activity

Practice Questions

1. Which of these is NOT a good way to improve writing style through grammar?
    a. Alternating among different sentence structures
    b. Using fewer words instead of unnecessary words
    c. Consistently using one-subject and one-verb sentences
    d. Writing in the active voice more than passive voice

2. Of the following statements, which is most accurate about topic sentences?
    a. They are always first in a paragraph.
    b. They are always last in a paragraph.
    c. They are only found once in every essay.
    d. They are explicit or may be implicit.

3. Which of the following is considered criteria for a good paragraph topic sentence?
    a. Clear
    b. Subtle
    c. Lengthy
    d. Ambiguous

4. "We don't go out as much because babysitters, gasoline, and parking is expensive." Which grammatical error does this sentence demonstrate?
    a. It contains a misplaced modifier.
    b. It lacks subject-verb agreement.
    c. It introduces a dangling participle.
    d. It does not have a grammar error.

5. Which of the following versions of a sentence has correct pronoun-antecedent agreement?
    a. Every student must consult their advisor first.
    b. All students must talk with their advisors first.
    c. All students must consult with his advisor first.
    d. Every student must consult their advisors first.

6. Which version of this sentence is grammatically correct?
    a. Give it to Shirley and I.
    b. Both Choices *C* and *D*.
    c. Give it to Shirley and me.
    d. Give it to me and Shirley.

7. What parts of speech are modified by adjectives?
    a. Verbs
    b. Nouns
    c. Pronouns
    d. Both Choices *B* and *C*

8. What part(s) of speech do adverbs modify?
   a. Verbs
   b. Adverbs
   c. Adjectives
   d. All of the above

9. What accurately reflects expert advice for beginning writers regarding topic sentences?
   a. They should use topic sentences in every two to three paragraphs.
   b. They should vary topic sentence positioning in paragraphs.
   c. They should include a topic sentence in every paragraph.
   d. They should make each topic sentence broad and general.

10. Being familiar with English words such as *claustrophobia, photophobia, arachnophobia, hydrophobia, acrophobia,* etc. could help a reader who is unfamiliar with the origin determine that the Greek *phobos* means which of these?
   a. Love
   b. Fear
   c. Hate
   d. Know

11. Which of the following English words is derived from a Greek source?
   a. Move
   b. Motor
   c. Moron
   d. Mobile

12. Homophones are defined as which of these?
   a. They have the same sounds.
   b. They have the same spelling.
   c. They have the same meaning.
   d. They have the same roots.

13. The word *tear,* pronounced one way, means a drop of eye fluid; pronounced another way, it means to rip. What is this type of word called?
   a. A homograph
   b. A heteronym
   c. A homonym
   d. Both *A* and *B*

14. Which of these words is considered a plural?
   a. Cactus
   b. Bacteria
   c. Criterion
   d. Elf

15. Which of these words has an irregular plural that is the same as its singular form?
   a. Louse
   b. Goose
   c. Mouse
   d. Moose

16. Of the following words with irregular plurals, which one has a plural ending *most* different from those of the others?
    a. Ox
    b. Child
    c. Person
    d. Woman

17. Which of the following sentences uses the apostrophe(s) correctly?
    a. Please be sure to bring you're invitation to the event.
    b. All of your friends' invitations were sent the same day.
    c. All of your friends parked they're cars along the street.
    d. Who's car is parked on the street leaving it's lights on?

18. Of the following, which word is spelled correctly?
    a. Wierd
    b. Forfeit
    c. Beleive
    d. Concieve

19. Which of these words has the correct spelling?
    a. Insolent
    b. Irrelevent
    c. Independant
    d. Indispensible

20. Exceptions and variations in rules for capitalization are accurately reflected in which of these?
    a. *Congress* is capitalized and so is *Congressional.*
    b. *Constitution* is capitalized as well as *Constitutional.*
    c. *Caucasian* is capitalized, but *white* referring to race is not.
    d. *African-American* and *Black* as a race are both capitalized.

21. Which of the following statements is true about the Oxford comma?
    a. It is the first comma in a s eries of three or more items.
    b. It is the last comma in a series before *or*, or before *and.*
    c. It is any comma separating items in series of three or more.
    d. It is frequently omitted because it does not serve a purpose.

22. In the following sentence, which version has the correct punctuation?
    a. Delegates attended from Springfield; Illinois, Alamo; Tennessee, Moscow; Idaho, and other places.
    b. Delegates attended from Springfield Illinois, Alamo Tennessee, Moscow Idaho, and other places.
    c. Delegates attended from Springfield, Illinois; Alamo, Tennessee; Moscow, Idaho; and other places.
    d. Delegates attended from Springfield, Illinois, Alamo, Tennessee, Moscow, Idaho, and other places.

23. Of the following phrases, which correctly applies the rules for hyphenation?
    a. Finely-tuned
    b. Family owned
    c. Friendly looking
    d. Fraudulent-ID claim

24. What is the rule for using quotation marks with a quotation inside of a quotation?
    a. Single quotation marks around the outer quotation, double quotation marks around the inner one
    b. Double quotation marks to enclose the outer quotation and also to enclose the inner quotation
    c. Single quotation marks that enclose the outer quotation as well as the inner quotation
    d. Double quotation marks around the outer quotation, single quotation marks around the inner one

25. Which of the following phrases correctly uses apostrophes?
    a. Dennis and Pam's house
    b. Dennis's and Pam's house
    c. Dennis' and Pam's house
    d. Dennis's and Pam house

26. To make irregular plural nouns possessive, which of these correctly applies the rule?
    a. Geeses' honks
    b. Childrens' toys
    c. Teeths' enamel
    d. Women's room

27. Which of the following is a writing technique recommended for attaining sentence fluency?
    a. Varying the endings of sentences
    b. Making sentence lengths uniform
    c. Using consistent sentence rhythm
    d. Varying sentence structures used

28. Among elements of an effective paragraph, the element of coherence is reflected by which of these?
    a. Focus on one main point throughout
    b. The use of logical and verbal bridges
    c. A sentence identifying the main idea
    d. Data, examples, illustrations, analysis

Answer Explanations

1. C: Good ways to improve writing style through grammatical choices include alternating among simple, complex, compound, and compound-complex sentence structures (Choice *A*) to prevent monotony and ensure variety; using fewer words when more words are unnecessary (Choice *B*); NOT writing all simple sentences with only one subject and one verb each (Choice *C*); and writing in the active voice more often than in the passive voice (Choice *D*). Active voice uses fewer words and also emphasizes action more strongly.

2. D: The topic sentence in a paragraph may be stated explicitly, or it may only be implied (Choice *D*), requiring the reader to infer what the topic is rather than identify it as an overt statement. The topic sentence of a paragraph is often at or near the beginning, but not always (Choice *A*). Some topic sentences are at the ends of paragraphs, but not always (Choice *B*). There is more than one topic sentence in an essay, especially if the essay is built on multiple paragraphs (Choice *C*).

3. A: Criteria for a good paragraph topic sentence include clarity, emphasis rather than subtlety (Choice *B*), brevity rather than length (Choice *C*), and straightforwardness rather than ambiguousness (Choice *D*).

4. B: The sentence lacks subject-verb agreement. Three nouns require plural "are," not singular "is." A misplaced modifier (Choice *A*) is incorrectly positioned, modifying the wrong part. For example, in Groucho Marx's famous joke, "One morning I shot an elephant in my pajamas. How he got into my pajamas I don't know" (*Animal Crackers,* 1930), he refers in the second sentence to the misplaced modifier in the first. A dangling participle (Choice *C*) leaves a verb participle hanging by omitting the subject it describes; e.g. "Walking down the street, the house was on fire."

5. B: Choice *A* lacks pronoun-antecedent agreement: "Every student" is singular but "their" is plural. Choice *B* correctly combines plural "All students" with plural "their advisors." Choice *C* has plural "All students" but singular "his advisor." Choice *D* has singular "Every student" but plural "their advisors."

6. B: When compounding subjects by adding nouns including proper nouns (names) to pronouns, the pronoun's form should not be changed by the addition. Since "Give it to me" is correct, not "Give it to I," we would not write "Give it to Shirley and I" (Choice *A*). "Shirley" and "me" are correct in either position in Choices *C* and *D*. "Give it to" requires an object. Only "me," "us," "him," "her," and "them" can be objects; "I," "we," "he," "she," and "they" are used as subjects, but never as objects.

7. D: Adjectives modify nouns (Choice *B*) or pronouns (Choice *C*) by describing them. For example, in the phrase "a big, old, red house," the noun "house" is modified and described by the adjectives "big," "old," and "red." Adjectives do not modify verbs (Choice *A*); adverbs do.

8. D: Adverbs modify verbs (Choice *A*), other adverbs (Choice *B*), or adjectives (Choice *C*). For example, in "She slept soundly," the verb is "slept" and the adverb modifying it is "soundly." In "He finished extremely quickly," the adverb "extremely" modifies the adverb "quickly." In "She was especially enthusiastic," the adverb "especially" modifies the adjective "enthusiastic."

9. C: Experts should advise students/beginning writers to include a topic sentence in every paragraph. Although professional writers do not always do this, beginners should, to learn how to write good topic sentences and paragraphs, rather than include a topic sentence in only every second or third paragraph (Choice *A*). Although experienced writers can also vary the positioning of topic sentences within paragraphs, experts advise new/learning writers to start paragraphs with topic sentences (Choice *B*). A topic sentence should be narrow and restricted, not broad and general (Choice *D*).

10. B: *Phobos* means "fear" in Greek. From it, English has derived the word *phobia*, meaning an abnormal or exaggerated fear; and a multitude of other words ending in -*phobia*, whose beginnings specify the object of the fear, as in the examples given. Another ubiquitous English word part deriving from Greek is *phil* as a prefix or suffix, meaning love (Choice *A*), such as *philosophy, hydrophilic, philanthropist,* and *philharmonic*. The Greek word for hate (Choice *C*) is *miseo,* found in English words like *misogyny* and *misanthrope*. The Greek word meaning wise or knowledge (Choice *D*) is *sophos,* found in English *sophisticated* and *philosophy*.

11. C: The English word *moron* is derived from the Greek *mor-* meaning dull or foolish. *Sophomore* also combines *soph* from Greek *sophos,* meaning wise, with *mor*—i.e. literally "wise fool." The words *move* (Choice *A*), *motor* (Choice *B*), *mobile* (Choice *D*), and many others are all derived from the Latin *mot-* or *mov-*, from the Latin words *movere,* to move and *motus,* motion.

12. A: Homophones are words that are pronounced the same way, but are spelled differently and have different meanings. For example, *lax* and *lacks* are homophones. Words spelled the same (Choice *B*) but with different meanings are homographs. Words with the same meaning (Choice *C*) are synonyms, which are spelled and pronounced differently.

13. D: Words that are spelled the same way are homographs (Choice *A*); if they are pronounced differently, they are heteronyms (Choice *B*). The example given fits both definitions. But homonyms (Choice *C*) are spelled the same way (i.e. homographs) AND also pronounced the same way (i.e. homophones), NOT differently. Therefore, Choices *A* and *B* both correctly describe *tear,* but Choice *C* does not.

14. B: Bacteria is considered a plural word. The singular word for "bacteria" is "bacterium." Cactus, criterion, and elf are all considered singular words, making Choices *A, C,* and *D* incorrect.

15. D: *Moose* is both the singular and plural form of the word. Other words that do not change from singular to plural include *deer, fish,* and *sheep*. *Louse* (Choice *A*) has an irregular plural, but it is *lice,* not the same as the singular. *Goose* (Choice *B*) has the irregular plural *geese,* also not the same as the singular. *Mouse* (Choice *C*), like *louse,* has the irregular plural *mice,* also different from its singular form.

16. C: The irregular plural of *ox* (Choice *A*) is *oxen*. The irregular plural of *child* (Choice *B*) is *children*. The irregular plural of *woman* (Choice *D*) is *women*. These irregular plurals all end in –*en*. However, *person* (Choice *C*) has the irregular plural of *people,* which has a different ending than the others. It can also be pluralized as *persons;* but this is a regular plural, not an irregular one.

17. B: The plural possessive noun *friends'* is correctly punctuated with an apostrophe following the plural -*s* ending. *Friend's* would indicate a singular possessive noun, i.e. belonging to one friend. *Friends* would indicate a plural noun not possessing anything. In Choice *A*, the second-person possessive is *your,* NOT "you're," a contraction of "you are." In Choice *C*, the third-person plural possessive is *their,* NOT "they're," a contraction of "they are." There are two errors in Choice *D*. The first possessive is *whose,* NOT "who's," a contraction of "who is;" the second is *its,* NOT "it's," a contraction of "it is."

18. B: *Forfeit* is spelled correctly. Choice *A* is misspelled and should be *weird*. Choice *C* is misspelled and should be *believe*. Choice *D* is misspelled and should be *conceive*. Many people confuse the spellings of words with *ie* and *ei* combinations. Some rules that apply to most English words, with 22 exceptions, are: I before E except after C; except after C and before L, P, T, or V; when sounding like A as in weight; when sounding like I as in height; or when an *ei* combination is formed by a prefix or a suffix.

19. A: *Insolent* is correctly spelled. Many people misspell words that sound the same but are spelled differently by confusing the vowels *a, e,* and *i.* For example, Choice *B* is correctly spelled *irrelevant;* Choice *C* is correctly spelled *independent;* and the correct spelling of Choice *D* is *indispensable.* Confusion is increased by these variations: Choices *B* and *C* sound the same but end with *-ant* and *-ent,* respectively; and while Choice *D* ends with *-able,* other words like *irrepressible* and *gullible* correctly end with *-ible,* which is incorrect in *indispensable.*

20. C: While terms like *Caucasian* and *African-American* are capitalized, the words *white* (Choice *C*) and *black* (Choice *D*) when referring to race should NOT be capitalized. While the name *Congress* is capitalized, the adjective *congressional* should NOT be capitalized (Choice *A*). Although the name of the U.S. *Constitution* is capitalized, the related adjective *constitutional* is NOT capitalized (Choice *B*).

21. B: The Oxford comma is the last comma following the last item in a series and preceding the word *or* or *and.* It is NOT the first (Choice *A*), or any comma separating items in a series (Choice *C*) other than the last. While it is true that many people omit this comma, it is NOT true that it serves no purpose (Choice *D*): It can prevent confusion when series include compound nouns.

22. C: A city and its state should always be separated by a comma. When items in a series contain internal commas, they should be separated by semicolons. City and state are never separated by a semicolon (Choice *A*). The city and its state are never named without punctuation between them (Choice *B*). The reason it is incorrect to use all commas, both between each city and its state and also between city-state pairs (Choice *D*), is obvious: some of the names used can refer to multiple places, causing serious confusion without different punctuation marks to identify them.

23. D: One rule for using hyphens is to clarify meaning: without the hyphen in this phrase, a reader could interpret it to mean that the claim is fraudulent; the hyphen makes it clear that it is the ID that is fraudulent. Another rule is that adverbs with *–ly* endings are not hyphenated, so Choice *A* should be *finely tuned.* However, an additional rule is that adjectives with *–ly* endings are hyphenated; hence Choice *B* should be *family-owned* and Choice *C* should be *friendly-looking.*

24. D: The rule for writing a quotation with another quotation inside it is to use double quotation marks to enclose the outer quotation, and use single quotation marks to enclose the inner quotation. Here is an example: "I don't think he will attend, because he said, 'I am extremely busy.'" The correct usage is reversed in Choice *A.* Choices *B* and *C* are incorrect, as this would not distinguish one quotation from the other.

25. A: When two people are named and both possess the same object, the apostrophe-*s* indicating possession should be placed ONLY after the second name, NOT after both names, making Choices *B* and *C* incorrect. It is also incorrect to use the apostrophe-*s* after the first name instead of the second (Choice *D*).

26. D: Irregular plurals that do not end in *–s* are always made possessive by adding apostrophe-*s.* A common error people make is to add *–s*-apostrophe instead of vice versa, as in the other three choices. *Geese* (Choice *A*), *children* (Choice *B*) and *teeth* (Choice *C*) are already plural, so adding an *s* before the apostrophe constitutes a double plural. Adding the *–s* after the apostrophe (i.e. *geese's, children's,* and *teeth's*) correctly makes these plurals possessive.

27. D: Some writing techniques recommended for attaining sentence fluency include varying the beginnings of sentences, making Choice *A* incorrect; varying sentence lengths rather than making them all uniform, making Choice *B* incorrect; varying sentence rhythms rather than consistently using the same rhythm, making Choice *C* incorrect; and varying sentence structures (Choice *D*) among simple, compound, complex, and compound-complex.

28. B: Four elements of an effective paragraph are unity, coherence, a topic sentence, and development. Focusing on one main point throughout (Choice *A*) the paragraph reflects the element of unity. Using logical and verbal bridges (Choice *B*) between/across sentences reflects the element of coherence. A sentence identifying the main idea (Choice *C*) of the paragraph reflects the element of a topic sentence. Citing data, giving examples, including illustrations, and analyzing (Choice *D*) the topic all reflect the element of developing the paragraph sufficiently.

Photo Credits

Greetings!

First, we would like to give a huge "thank you" for choosing us and this study guide for your TEAS 6 exam. We hope that it will lead you to success on this exam and for your years to come.

Our team has tried to make your preparations as thorough as possible by covering all of the topics you should be expected to know. In addition, our writers attempted to create practice questions identical to what you will see on the day of your actual test. We have also included many test-taking strategies to help you learn the material, maintain the knowledge, and take the test with confidence.

We strive for excellence in our products, and if you have any comments or concerns over the quality of something in this study guide, please send us an email so that we may improve.

As you continue forward in life, we would like to remain alongside you with other books and study guides in our library. We are continually producing and updating study guides in several different subjects. If you are looking for something in particular, all of our products are available on Amazon. You may also send us an email!

Sincerely,
APEX Test Prep
info@apexprep.com

FREE

Free Study Tips DVD

In addition to the tips and content in this guide, we have created a FREE DVD with helpful study tips to further assist your exam preparation. **This FREE Study Tips DVD provides you with top-notch tips to conquer your exam and reach your goals.**

Our simple request in exchange for the strategy-packed DVD is that you email us your feedback about our study guide. We would love to hear what you thought about the guide, and we welcome any and all feedback—positive, negative, or neutral. It is our #1 goal to provide you with top quality products and customer service.

To receive your **FREE Study Tips DVD**, email freedvd@apexprep.com. Please put "FREE DVD" in the subject line and put the following in the email:

   a. The name of the study guide you purchased.

   b. Your rating of the study guide on a scale of 1-5, with 5 being the highest score.

   c. Any thoughts or feedback about your study guide.

   d. Your first and last name and your mailing address, so we know where to send your free DVD!

Thank you!

CPSIA information can be obtained
at www.ICGtesting.com
Printed in the USA
BVHW011353181021
619205BV00014B/307

9 781628 458060